4.4

LESSONS FROM YEARS OF CELIBACY

CANDALADA

For the inner child in us all.

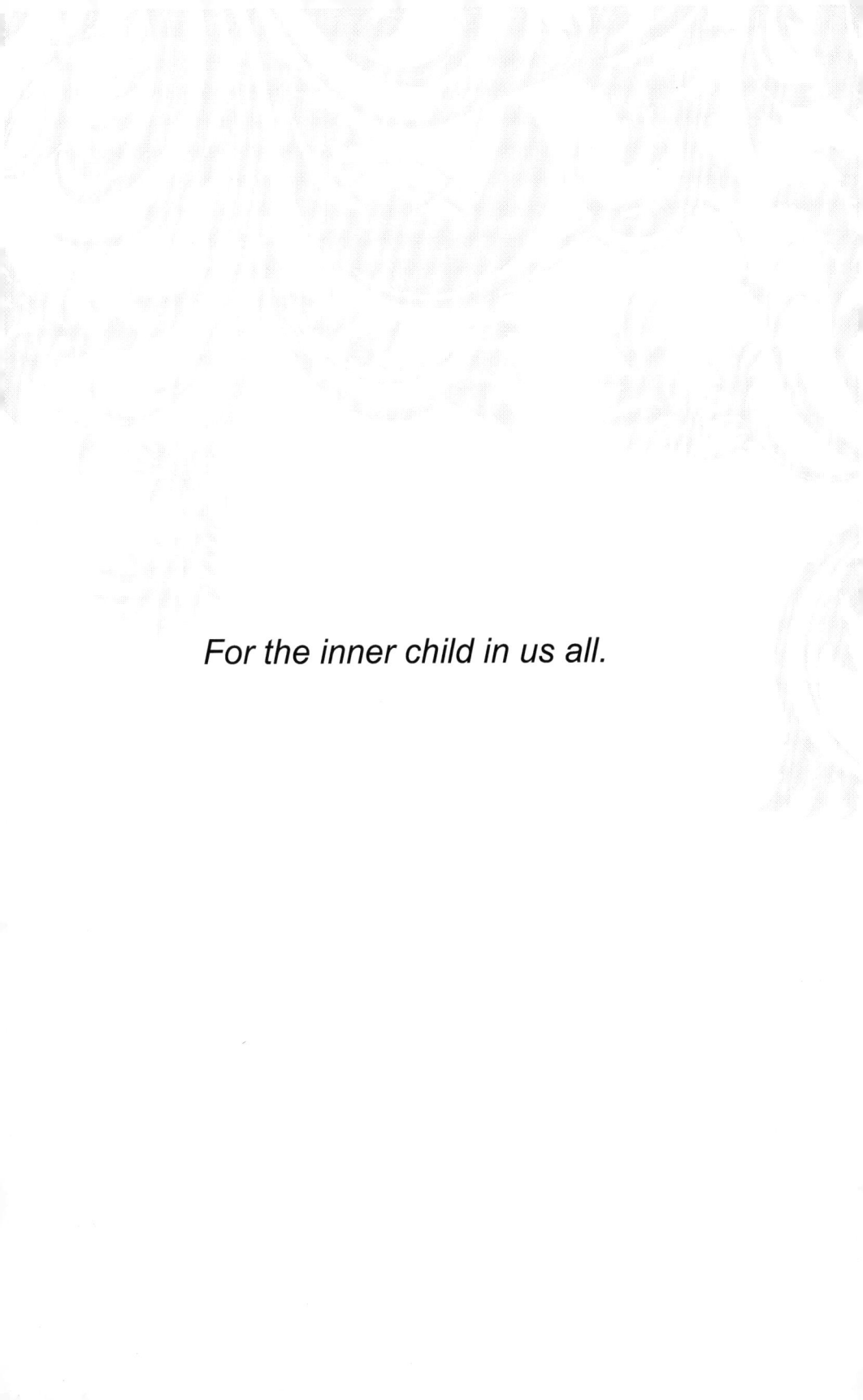

TABLE OF CONTENT

Introduction	1
Chapter 1	10
September 2018: The Dark Hole	10
The beginning of September	10
The end of September	14
April is for Issa 2019	20
August is for Me 2019	24
Chapter 2	26
September 2019: In the Nick of Time (One Year)	26
RAE2020	26
April is for Issa 2020	34
August is for Me 2020	36
August is for Me 2019	40
Chapter 3	42
September 2020: Chasing Waterfalls (Two Years)	42
Cascades Falls	43
Book Club	45
Winter	48
Triple Falls, Looking Glass, Dry Falls	52
April is for Issa 2021	55
August is for Me 2021	60
Chapter 4	62
September 2021: Superwoman (Three Years)	62
"Superwoman"	64
My Feelings in English	65
Winter	70
RAE2022	72
April is for Issa 2022	75
August is for Me 2023	83

Chapter 5 — 84
  September 2022-January 2023: Happy to Stupid (Four Years, Four Months) — 84
    Grandma's Birthday 2022 — 86

Chapter 6 — 102
  ShapeJanuary 27, 2023-September 27, 2023: Crash Out, Then Heal (Eight Months) — 102
    Dahlia — 111
    Rita — 117
    Hoodoo — 119
    Dahlia Session 2 — 122
    April is for Issa 2023 — 125
    Dahlia Session 3 — 132
    August is for Me 2023 — 144

Chapter 7 — 154
  September 2023-2024: The Year of the Rose — 154
    Dark Spiritual Baths Round 2 — 155
    White Spiritual Baths — 157
    Grandma's Birthday 2023 — 160
    The Year of Responsibility — 162
    Academic Advocacy for Prince Issa — 165
    RAE2024 — 167
    The Exorcism — 170
    April is for Issa 2024 — 174
    The Walkthrough — 179
    The Rose — 190

This Story is too Long. What are the Lessons? — 195
Conclusion — 197
4.4 Playlist — 200
Hymns and Spiritual — 200
4.4 Movies and Shows — 200

Acknowledgments	**203**
About the Author	**207**
Bibliography	**208**
Notes	**209**

INTRODUCTION

I checked the response *no* to the question "Are you sexually active?" for my annual physical for several years in my late thirties. How did I get there? The short answer is grief, sexual abuse, and regret. The long answers are in the detailed chapters of this book.

In my opinion, sex is a simple and complex act. It can bring pleasure and joy or pain and regret. Some variables that have affected my experience are age, relationship status, and emotional intelligence.

The early years of my sexual history were explorative and foolish because I started having sex when I was too young—high school, to be specific. I often wonder if my sexual exploration would have been delayed or prevented had I lived with my father during my high school years. I lived with both of my parents from birth to four years old. I lived with my dad from age four to nine and my mom from ten to adulthood. When I was fourteen and in the ninth grade, I lived in Brooklyn, New York; then from age fifteen and up (from tenth to twelfth grade and college) in Virginia. I don't remember the ability to think of a boy in my father's presence, not because he was threatening, but because I was very enamored with our bonding and adventures.

Before delving into my high school experience, I will reflect on the prerequisite, **middle school**. To get to Shellbank Junior High, I took the bus for forty-five minutes from East Fortieth Street to Sheepshead Bay for three years. That level of independence aged me a bit. It was normal to me and the other city kids. I clutch my pearls at the thought of sending my son, currently twelve years old, on the bus route I took at his age. During my long commute to school, I saw the usual things: nurses going to and from work and senior citizens reading books. I also saw unusual things: drug addicts and homeless people on the park benches, both dead and alive.

At the time, I did not have a great concept of what was age-appropriate for my peers and me. I knew I was not an adult, but I felt like one when I was outside of the house. The language I heard and used was obscene. The boys were more explicit in the use of the words fuck, bitch, and pussy. Popular phrases were, "Fuck you," "You a bitch," and "You a pussy." The boys were prideful in their mission to insult one another. Middle school is when I first started using the "f" word in the context of "Fuck this," "Fuck that," and "What the fuck?!" Boys went from invisible to visible. I had my first crush in sixth grade. He was still cute in eighth grade and became my first kiss!

High School was another planet where we all acted eighteen plus despite our lack of life experience, money, or job retention. High school was the first time I felt curious about how sex would feel. I soon learned it was painful and felt no pleasure from intercourse in high school. I learned that I liked being rubbed and touched, but penetration felt so uncomfortable and forbidden. Very regrettable times. My first grew up to be a gigolo. He currently has over ten children. We broke up three months after my first time; rumor had it he started sleeping with his cousin! This was a challenging first experience that left me feeling dumb and emotional. I do not know what I expected to happen. I cried a lot and never told any adults about it. My tenth and eleventh-grade boyfriend broke up with me at the end of the school year with no explanation. I thought everything was fine, and once summer hit, things were over. More tears. As a senior, I got a job at a sneaker store where I met my high school senior year and soon-to-be college boyfriend.

The **college** years of sex were hormonal and fun. I was not living with my parents. I was a young adult in a long-term and loving relationship. We dated for six years. In this relationship, I discovered pleasure. I experienced comfort; no more sneaking and hiding. Cuddling, foreplay, and sleepovers were new and exciting to me. It was in this relationship during my college years that I learned that everything I had done previously was a waste of time. Upon reflection, I risked pregnancy, life-threatening STDs, and emotional stability at the time when I was unemployed or, at best, making $5.15 an hour! I should have been shaping my creativity, improving my vocals, or playing a sport. My parents warned me that young relationships are dangerous and nonsensical, and I did not listen.

After college, I left my high school sweetheart and explored California. After one year, I returned to Virginia. Soon after, I entered my second-longest relationship to date and, toward the end of it, completed my Master's degree.

I had my son the following year of graduation. I created a confessional-style documentary, "41 Weeks In," about my pregnancy journey. The drama-filled story of my experience with my son's father, Mr. Sexy, is in my first book, *Beautiful Reject*. *Beautiful Reject* covers seven years of delusional dating from 2010 to 2015. Therefore, I am rolling right through all of those stories and getting closer to the part where sex stopped. Where did the sex stop? Why did the sex stop?

You may have noticed that 2010 to 2015 isn't quite seven years. What happened from 2015 to 2017? Why did I leave readers hanging like that? I left my readers to assume it took about two years to walk away from Classic Man. The Return of

Classic Man 2015 dragged on for a while, longer than I would like to admit publicly. There was a break of communication in 2016. However, my feelings for him interfered with and interrupted any attempts at sanity and normalcy in 2016. I was not ready to discuss 2016 and still unsure if I should write about it.

I spent 2016 in a brief but serious relationship with someone I had a plutonic twenty-year friendship with. He was very serious about me and immediately began discussing marriage. In exactly four weeks, I was pregnant from our first time being intimate. I was in shock. I could not believe it. Back then, when I told him I was writing my first book, he was opposed to the idea. Naturally, that only made me want to complete the book even more. However, it did create an unspoken protection I have put around my good relationships when writing about my story. There is a difference between the mistakes I've made and sharing so many details; it can subsequently ruin other people's lives.

The men who were good to me could honestly write a book about me, and I would be the villain. Sometimes I think the shitty dating experiences I have had are karma for the few good men I have left brokenhearted for some reason or another. The most similar thing about those breakups is that they never stemmed from arguments. They came from me thinking I could not achieve some of my goals if we remained together. The breakups came from fear and the predictive nature of thinking things won't end well. I learned years later that being predictive is a cognitive filter. Ending something that is not working is not the same as ending something you think won't work.

How did September 2016 end? It ended in abortion. I was being told and shown that I was loved, and my heart and mind did not trust it. What if it didn't work out? I would be a single mother of two! If I am happy, why am I still thinking about Classic Man? With all of those reservations, I couldn't bring myself to do it. I dealt with the shame of going back to my family and letting them know. I am not getting married and I am not having a baby. I didn't give anyone the reasons. I spent the rest of 2016 rebuilding my credit, becoming an adjunct professor, and crying. The friendship was damaged severely, and there wasn't much left to say.

In August 2017, I participated in a nonprofit event that provided hair services free of charge for back-to-school students. I met Mr. Suavemente at this event. He was tall with brown skin, curly hair, and an all-black outfit. He carried a gold briefcase and wore gold Foamposites to match. He had a gentle voice when he said, "Hello." I watched him work throughout the day, and eventually, he suggested we exchange numbers.

In the upcoming weeks, I received text messages with heart eyes and found myself smiling again. I thought he looked like a Ken doll. Perhaps we will call him Ken instead. We went on our first date shortly after meeting. I went back to his house afterward, we listened to music, had a few kisses, and I fell asleep in his arms. It seemed perfect.

Shortly after, he went on a trip. I was a little surprised to see his pic in Miami floating down my timeline because he didn't mention it. It was the beginning of our getting to know each other, so I didn't think much of it.

Once he returned, he told me he was home, and I responded that I missed him. He invited me to come over. I told him I had rollers in my hair. He convinced me he didn't care about the rollers and just wanted to see me. This night would change everything for me. We watched one episode of a show on Netflix, and as soon as the show was over, he leaned over and kissed me. It was very passionate, too passionate. He started pulling down my underwear.

I told him, "Wait, wait, I'm not ready." I moved my arms and tried to push him away. He pinned them down, said relax, and shoved it in. A single tear rolled down my cheek. I had a myriad of emotions. I felt paralyzed, no fight in me. I felt that since his body had already entered mine, what was the point?! I didn't moan; I didn't say encouraging phrases like, "Yes, this feels good" or "Don't stop," but I don't think he noticed. I lay there the rest of the night, certain and confused that I was raped by a very handsome man who was turned on by the word no.

In the following days, I expressed that I was uncomfortable with how the night unfolded. He blew off my complaints, continued to call me baby, and eventually asked to see me again. I talked myself out of believing that it was the nightmare that it was. I convinced myself that if I could date this handsome man, I wouldn't feel so terrible about our first time together.

He continued to treat me worse and worse. One time, when I leaned over to kiss him, he removed me from his body, lifted me, and placed me on the other side of the bed. Then he took a FaceTime from another woman and discussed their upcoming travel plans. I was outraged, and I left his house. My thought was that it must be nice to be strong and be able to move a woman when you don't want her to touch you, yet use those same hands to hold her down weeks prior. I felt so crazy and blamed myself for my decision to ever go over there. I felt it was too late to report the rape, and no one would believe me. They would focus on why I returned or maintained communication with my abuser.

Unfortunately, his story inspired me to create my first art show/ documentary screening. I created the concept of a documentary about men who look nice but have a rough past.

It was October 2017, and we were a few months out from the premier. Instead of throwing him out of my show and finding a replacement, I continued to work with him despite what I had gone through. We did photo and video shoots during October and November in preparation for the big day in February.

This is one point in my life where I didn't fight back. As a person who is so spunky and all about justice, it appalled me that I didn't take immediate official action. Sending angry texts after the fact solved nothing. Continuing to give him a platform to be showcased fed his ego and empowered him. This is the first time I put someone who hurt me in the position to hurt others. Why? Why? Why!!!

Dismayed in myself, I was compelled to research and blog about my findings. While that was informative, it did not make me feel any better. Currently, I go to the range regularly and swore to myself that if anything like this should ever happen again, I'm willing to take a murder charge because filing a report isn't enough. I must overcompensate for the missed opportunity to be brave and report the abuse in September 2017.

In December 2017, I reconnected with a guy from high school (the fireman) through social media. We went on a coffee date and later celebrated his birthday together. Although I still communicated with Ken about the upcoming show, I was disgusted with him. I spent my time with the fireman, who was relaxed and, at the time, focused on me being comfortable and pleased. He made an Olympic sport out of eating me out and made sure I was dripping wet before whispering in my ear, "Can I put it in?" or "May I feel you?" This was the complete opposite of what I had recently gone through and I liked it.

The year 2018 was extreme highs and lows. I premiered the art show/documentary known as Rappers and Entrepreneurs

(RAE) on February 11, which was a great accomplishment; I was fired earlier that month on the second of February, which was a great disappointment. I used money from my tax returns to fund the show, and once that money was depleted, I had no idea where the next dollar was coming from.

Forty-four people attended RAE2018, and at least thirty-five were there to see Ken. He drew a crowd, but it would have probably been better to stand in an empty room than continue to work with and be exposed to him. Noticeably, the man he arrived with was gay, and many of the attendees were gay. He certainly never mentioned he was bisexual, but judging by how roughly he handled me, I think he would have preferred if I was a man. I kept my composure that evening and opened no discussion about it. My goal was to make it through the evening and break even and I did.

My mom's cancer came back in 2016, and her condition worsened. This made it tough to focus on work. I found myself seeking comfort in the arms of men who had no plans to love me. Casual dating requires a carefree attitude that I couldn't access. I was in a panicked state with no safe place. I was in a pattern of isolation, followed by attracting men looking for company and nothing more. It was a diminishing and seemingly helpless time. February 2018 to September 2018 carried the weight of functioning while waiting for the worst thing to happen.

By late 2018, the fireman and I had already gone through a series of breakups. Although he laid it on thick in the beginning, he was not able to maintain that after he returned to work. When we reconnected, he was on vacation, and apparently, our experience made the vacation/staycation interesting. Once he started not calling as consistently, I would complain. One time, he ignored my text asking about the change in behavior, and I lost it. His response to that snap was to ignore me more. The almost final straw was that he kept saying he valued our friendship and didn't even care about the sex, which was super annoying. It was really a nice way of saying I see no future with you because he definitely cared about the sex. I would get quiet, and he would reach out and ask, "How are you today?" "Did you eat today?" and text on holidays.

In September 2018, I reached the highest level of stress from losing my mother on September 2. I saw her last heartbeat, and I haven't been the same since. I kept busy between funeral arrangements and renovating my mom's home. The family home known as 3421.

September 2018, September 2018, September 2018

CHAPTER 1

SEPTEMBER 2018

THE DARK HOLE

The beginning of September:

I had never witnessed the end of a human life until September 2, 2018. It is the single most helpless feeling there is. My mom's passing took place on a holiday weekend, five days after my thirty-sixth birthday (August 28, 2018). I remember not wanting to celebrate my life while she was losing hers. Food had no taste, and night had no sleep.

I started looking for hospice on August 23, secured one by August 27, and she transitioned on September 2. This week had to be the longest week in history. Several decisions had to be made in a small amount of time. I moved Mom downstairs to make it easy for the visitors and doctors to see her. I put up a curtain in the hallway so there would be some level of privacy for her and give visitors a moment to mentally prepare for what they were about to see instead of seeing her in a hospital bed as soon as they came in the door. There were many friends and family this week, yet I still felt alone.

The most challenging part of this process was my mom becoming nonverbal. Her last words to me were, "Candice." She looked at me and said my name as I helped her into her new hospice bed. I still have trouble hearing my name these days; Candy and Candalada go over smoothly, but something happens to me every time I hear my name.

Within these six days, I desperately hoped my mom could hear me and was satisfied with what I was saying. I transferred her retirement assets to her account and paid the mortgage and utilities. I had the garden in the front done and the backyard cleaned because it looked like a jungle. I reported each improvement, hoping it made her comfortable enough to let go. I wanted her to know I was capable of handling the things she usually did.

The most unexpected thing that happened during that week. On August 28, a mom from a shelter where I volunteered my hair services texted me to say she needed help. She and her kids were outside with no place to stay, and their items had been kicked out of storage because they could not pay the bills. I left the house to pick her and her sons up. They were surrounded by bags and boxes outside a storage center a few exits away. We drove back to my house quietly. They stayed for two days. This was not the best timing; however, I did what I could while thinking, damn, life can get pretty tough, and if you don't figure it out, your kids will be dragged into the harsh reality with you.

August 28 was also the day my mom's end-of-life medicine arrived. The doctor explained how to put it in apple sauce and warned me that she would go from speaking rarely to not speaking. Before she went nonverbal, I remember my mom kept saying that she was lost, and I interpreted that as her looking for her placement on the other side. Giving her the medicine that was supposed to help her with the pain she was experiencing still made me feel like I was hurting her. I eventually relinquished this duty to the nurse because I was too broken up.

Something I am grateful for and astonished by is the accuracy of the hospice nurse and my mom's doctors. Her oncologist told me it would be ninety days, and it was exactly that. The hospice nurse told me when to sleep. She said, "You will not miss anything; take this night of rest." When I woke up in the morning, she said, "It will be today; you have a few hours." In the last twenty minutes, she said, "It will be anytime now; all that want to be present should gather."

I couldn't believe that all that transpired would boil down to this last twenty minutes. I held Mom's hand. My sister lay beside her, and a family member prayed while Whitney Houston's "I Will Always Love You" played. Two of my aunts were there. My uncle was there. My grandpa was there. He was weeping. Mom's chest went up then down and never came back up again. My dad called. He couldn't hear through my tears, and in pure frustration, I dropped the phone. That was it. My mommy was gone.

I spent the next few hours in my room listening to music. I read that it is best not to watch the body be removed from the home, so I followed that advice. I slept with my sister that night, and we didn't say much. My son spent the evening with my aunt, and she called to say he had fallen ill and was vomiting all night. I was sure that his body was rejecting the fact that his grandma was gone, and he was terribly sad.

September 2 to 16 created the greatest divide between my family and me. "What do you need help with?" wasn't a question I heard. There was a suggestion made for a specific preacher, but I didn't say yes, and that was the beginning of World War 3. At the end of it all, there was not one card or check from those with suggestions. The next showdown was about how and when I cleaned, repaired, and restored the estate.

The most outrageous statement I heard was that I was not grieving, and her memorial was one of my promotional events. This backlash came because the service was not held in a church. There was no viewing, and my mom's body was not present at the memorial. Not having a body present was a request from my grandfather. This type of service is not traditional by Guyanese standards.

There is a lot of speculation on why things became so chaotic at the time. All I can say is that all the shit-talking had me doubting myself as a daughter. I felt unloved and abandoned because I wouldn't do what others told me to do at thirty-six. I was fed up with all of it, and I wished very much that I could die as well and leave them all since I was such a fucking problem. Luckily, I found my way to therapy. Session by session, I learned how to reject the negative statements I had started to internalize and believe. When I was able, I addressed the people that stressed me out the most—my aunts and my sister—and attempted to move on.

Unfortunately, disgruntled feelings would reappear for years to come clear into 2024. Handling never-ending resentment was challenging. The key thing that has changed was becoming sure of who I am. I am the first-born daughter of Shelly Browne. It is my birthright as long as I am coherent to tend to her affairs and legacy. If ever I should fall, next in line is my brother, and if he was unable, my sister. That is generally how it goes when there is no husband or partner to shield this burden from the children. I watched this natural order play out time and time again while growing up, and somehow, when it was my turn, everyone seemed really confused about the natural order.

One thing I do not like about my South American/Caribbean culture is that age seems to trump everything, and you can get stuck in a vortex where you are permanently viewed as a child. This comes with a lack of respect and an instinct to override and challenge every decision you make. I suspect if I were fifty, things would have been different.

I had one immediate and uncomplicated reconciliation with my Aunty Roxy. We screamed it out and resolved things. I held her on a pillar; she was the only adult to apologize to me instead of rationalizing. It was like an instant diffusion as we spoke on the phone just moments after the unruliest declaration I have ever made, which took place on the evening of my mother's memorial. After viewing the shenanigans all day, I couldn't stand it anymore. I displayed no decorum and no understanding as I was screaming out raw and unfiltered feelings.

Since then, my aunt and I have been growing at a rate that others can't catch up with. I am grateful for this rebirth because our relationship is better than before. I am currently learning a lot from her. She is the glue of the family, always hosting parties and showing up for others. She is emotionally intelligent in most cases. When it comes to my cousins, you can forget it. She will always defend her children; I learned that from her and do the same.

The end of September:

On September 23, 2018, one week after Mom's memorial, the fireman texted me.

"Hey, Candy. I found your earrings."

What earrings was he talking about? We went back and forth on IG about when I should get them or if he would bring them to me. We finally decided that I would go and get the earrings.

I entered the basement; it was dark, and the TV was on. He walked to his dresser, slid the earrings into the palm of his hand, then opened his hand. "Here they are."

I stared at them for a minute because these earrings belonged to my mother. They were not made of expensive material; they were cute, fun, iridescent cubes. It still made me heartsick to think of her. My entire mood changed. Immediately, I felt a headache coming on, and I wanted to lie down. He gave me hugs around my back, and that was very comforting. What wasn't so comforting was him placing my hand on his private parts. Of all days, this was not a day I was interested in servicing another person. A simple cuddle would be more than enough for me.

He continued to kiss me, and I didn't push him away, but I was wondering where this was all headed. I think he picked up on the fact that I wasn't my usual self. He showered me with kisses everywhere. Then he got on his knees and proceeded to lick and slurp me like an icy from 7-Eleven. Even with this outstanding performance, I wasn't motivated to return the favor or go further. He asked me if I was ready, and I said *no*. He responded by proceeding to kiss and lick me more, and then he asked again if he could feel me. I said yes but knew this would be our last time together.

It came over me that for some, I represent sexual pleasure, and nothing, I mean nothing, turns that desire off. This includes extreme life circumstances, death, mourning—nothing. I decided I no longer wanted to be in the presence of men. They were going to find a way for me to make them feel better, even on the days when I needed consoling and not sex.

He wasn't aggressive, and he wasn't disrespectful. Given my history and recent events, it would have been nice for him to be more intuitive, but I didn't have it in me to try to teach this lesson because he would know better for someone he loved. This is the consequence of not being loved but still being in someone's bed. Thus, the rendezvous had to end.

I made no big declarations or statements. I went home and minded my business for the rest of the year. For that, I am proud. He reached out here and there and also invited me over again. I politely declined and told him I was tired of situationships and needed more out of life. He is married now; looks like he figured it out. The ratio of men who get married right after meeting me is mind-boggling.

I finished out September with a bright patch of teal hair. I chose this color to represent ovarian cancer. I wore my mom's Hair Therapy hoodie, the one she cut down the middle to give her air for the hot flashes.

In November, things with the family at large were still estranged, but my immediate family and I kept striving to be productive and reinvent ourselves. On November 3, my sister released her first book and had her first show, Counter Point. My dad was in town on November 5, and we celebrated his sixtieth birthday with a helicopter ride. My grandpa was in town all of November; he took me to breakfast and bought me the book, *Becoming*, which meant so much to me. On November 15, my son started guitar lessons. In the moments of silence, I hurled myself into home improvement, even having a contractor work on the floors on Thanksgiving morning.

Unknowingly, this November marked a turning point by setting a template for the future. My sister continued her professional photography career. My dad and I went on to create many new travel experiences. In the coming years, I would drive to Long Island and maintain my relationship with my grandpa as he got older. Issa went from a kid who could not read music to a sixth-year guitar student in 2024.

In late November 2018, I lost the bracelet with my name on it that my dad bought me for completing my undergrad studies. I had it for twelve years. The loss of it is one of the greatest mysteries of this year and another reason I hated this year so much. I always thought of that bracelet as a gentle reminder of what my dad would do. It was a reminder to take the path with less gasoline in any given situation. My dad once explained to me that you can use water or gasoline in any situation and asked why I chose gasoline most times.

I also would look at my bracelet when I wanted to shift my thoughts to the future. Thinking of the future was the easiest way to escape the pain or stress of the present. It kept me motivated and moving. The downfall was that sometimes, my reactions and thoughts about what was happening in the present were delayed because I was distracted. Reflecting on what happened and sharing my delayed thoughts or emotions upsets some people. They often are more concerned with why I didn't say those things right away than what I am complaining about. Many repeat the phrase, "time is relative," and throw the concept out the window when it comes to delayed reactions. In that case, time is apparently immediate.

I officially lost my mind in 2018. Not in the way that you may think. The visualization of my mind. Often, when I close my eyes at night, the background looks black, and the writing looks blue, similar to the simulations that you see in *Wreck-It Ralph 2*. There are tons of windows open and different options and paths to take in the upcoming years. It was in these dreams that I saw a way to create Hair Therapy, a way to make it to California, a path to come home, and a path to take care of my mom, and now it was gone. My mind and the bracelet left at the same time. As a result, December was pitch black. When I closed my eyes, I saw nothing. I felt no present, and I saw no future. I was officially suspended in time. Paused.

I remember very few things about December 2018. While awake, I spent my days gutting my mom's kitchen, preparing for its renovation. I spoke to no one on Christmas Day. I thought about people being in their matching pajamas, making hot cocoa, and sitting by the fireplace as depicted on TV versus my reality of laying in bed where the only person checking on my well-being was six years old. I went to see Bumblebee with my son on Christmas evening, which brought me great joy. January does not even have a documented photo to help me piece together what happened.

February was eventful. The undercurrent was that my heart was broken. The same old heartbreak from Classic Man that I piled several relationship attempts on top of was then amplified by grief, sexual abuse, and not being able to find a place where my heart and body were comfortable. Sometimes, I wish we had been issued several hearts to deal with different issues. We are issued one, and it's supposed to process emotions plus get blood everywhere in the body. Seems like an impossible task. (I know emotions are handled in the brain; for the sake of imagination and artistry, let me have this.)

On the surface, I smiled and went where I was invited with lots of makeup. If it wasn't for my subposts, an outsider looking in could assume I was one hundred percent happy. I attended a Total Wine alcohol education class. I went to the movies to see *My Online Valentine,* an independent film, and was dazzled by Blue Kimble. On Valentine's Day, I had lunch with a former client turned family. We ate healthy; she gave me some advice, chocolate, and a candle. The next day, I had an opportunity to attend a backstage Erykah Badu concert. I listened to some live loud music, one of my favorite pastimes. I gifted Erykah my first product, The Perfect Head Tie, which was such a big deal to me. It was cold that night and that solo ride to Baltimore was daunting, but the outcome of the evening was worth it.

February was also the month when I returned to doing hair. The accounts were empty, and I needed to earn income. This fiscal deprivation is what fueled the promotion of my head ties and styling hair at home. I went through my phone and checked messages that had been abandoned for months. I was not aware that my new iPhone separated texts from unsaved numbers. After issuing a few apologies, I was doing locs, retwists, and haircuts.

Just like that, I was rolling into six months of no physical sexual contact. It didn't feel like six months because my relationship with time was distorted. Sometimes, one day felt like a year, and a month felt like a day. While my heart longed for someone who wasn't available, my body was content being safe and rested.

In March, I was invited to California under the pretense of attending the National Association for the Advancement of Colored People (NAACP) Awards. I got my hair done, bought a new ball gown, and was on my way. When we got there, a ticket was only issued to my friend. I was left on the outskirts of the red carpet, and guess who walked by—my movie crush, Blue Kimble. He looked at me and smiled. My day was made. I was still pissed, but for a moment, I thought of how entertainers can appear out of reach when they are only a flight or a brief introduction away.

My friend went on to see Chloe and Halle Bailey and Viola Davis. What drove the nail in my coffin was when he saw Jay-Z accept the NAACP President's Award. To say I was disappointed was an understatement. I am a huge Jay-Z fan and a Brooklyn native, and that was not a moment that can be duplicated. After the Fiftieth NAACP Awards, we were also rejected from the after-party at the Roosevelt Hotel.

The coordinator overpromised and underdelivered. The box office was unmoved by our story, familiar with the coordinator but fed up with her. Her name had no merit there. The hotel bouncer stated that only VIP tickets to the awards were given after-party entry. I passed several familiar faces on my way back down the stairs and out of the hotel. That day, I felt like Cinderella who hadn't gone to the ball in a carriage.

As the attendees arrived in Rolls Royces, I walked back to my hotel defeated after doing a two-step to "Candy" by Cameo for Instagram. On Instagram, I didn't share this depressing story. I shared my look of the evening with a smile. My friend apologized for the inconvenience, and I spent the rest of the trip catching up with my Cali cousins and trying to forget about the ordeal. I missed the check-in for my flight because I went to Manhattan Beach to get pizza. Luckily, the attendant was able to switch my seat to the next flight with no additional expense to me.

April is for Issa 2019

Like August of every year, my world stops for my son in April. His birthday is on the fifth. After his first birthday, I vowed to keep our birthdays very personal. The pressure of cooking food and tending to other adults was too much for me. When Issa turned two, three, four, five, and six, I took him for a cupcake. In 2017, when he turned six, a car full of us headed to Alexandria for a cupcake for Issa at high noon. He was dressed in the cutest black outfit with white speckles on it. The front of the shirt said, "Always Laugh Loudly." Later that evening, the entire extended family came to my house and decided to go bowling. Issa thought it was a party that I put together for him. There was actually a death that my aunts and cousins were in town for, a completely unplanned coincidence. I didn't burst the excitement he had that day.

This year, I made a plan to take him to The St. James, a fancy new sports center that opened near my house. We visited the play center, Super, Awesome & Amazing. He played with whatever kids were there, and we went to lunch at the restaurant upstairs. His hair was immaculate, and I took tons of pictures. I was completely satisfied with our outing. Knock, knock—It's Aunty Roxy and my cousin. Hi, we are taking Issa out to play laser tag. He had the time of his life with his cousin. Cheers to another surprise I didn't plan that went well. My aunty clearly saw how isolated we had become and used her aunty magic to create a family-inclusive celebration.

April is always a tricky time. It is the anniversary of being a mom. Each year, I look at how much my son has grown, and I can't believe he went from being the tiniest little veggie nugget to what he is. The elephant in the room is that his father is not there. Year after year. It is an emptiness I cannot fill and a sadness. This is possibly an underlying reason why I started the intimate birthday tradition, so I can pay close attention to my son and make sure I am personally showering him instead of running around like a chicken with my head cut off catering to others.

I was dreaming and hustling big in May. I worked on my newsletter tirelessly and spent time with my favorite clients. I was posting every day about my head tie and still in my feelings from time to time over Classic Man. It would go from casual conversation to me lashing out. It was just inevitable. I thought to myself, God hates me. I have no money. I am getting rejection emails left and right from ABC, Warner Brothers, and any other cool media job I tried to secure. All of my selfies showed smiles and a mother-and-son bond.

My IG stories were all about how marriages are bullshit and do not let men play in your face. I was so unhappy. I longed for a shoulder to lean on, literally, not digitally. I was grappling with dwindling finances, my products not selling, my mom being gone, and my person of choice being taken. I listened to the DVSN albums September 5 ("With Me," "Too Deep," "Do it Well," "Hallucinations," "The Line")—The Morning After ("Think About Me," "Body Smile," "Nuh Time/Tek Time") on an endless loop. I did expressive dances at home and lay in the dark as early as 6 p.m. most nights. So much was happening, but the results were unimpressive.

One thing I didn't let up on as summer approached was being sexy. There was zero visible indication that I was going through anything. My teal had faded from light green into grey, so I got really creative with my next look. Mini dresses with a trench coat paired with high buns and a bang. Chinese bobs with Bob Marley shirts and leather pants. Blue wig with the black sundress.

My runway looks could not save me from those damn emails. This month, it was Amazon Web Services. My friend tried her best to put me on, and the rejections flew back about as fast as she could recommend me. Public Sector Editor and Writer, Content Manager, Senior Manager Editorial, Senior Internal Communications Specialist—no, no, no, and no.

In the meantime, I traveled to clients, styled hair for proms, styled hair for weddings, I did locs, weaves, braids, twists, and rod sets—everyone looked fetching. I was grateful to spend some time with my mentor, who hired me to do some hair for a wedding. I admitted to him over dinner that I had no idea what was next. He gave me two pieces of advice: Know what you want to be and find the name of it—the exact title. Don't stop.

"I have seen all that you do, and if you keep going, something is bound to happen. Others will see, and it will take you somewhere good."

July was wild. I fell off my bed trying to take something off the ceiling. I posted online that I fell and needed help after calling my nearest family members. A friend came by with a bag of ice and helped me. I went through it with my siblings, who chastised me for running out of money and trying to find solutions to keep everything afloat. This month, I wore a huge Crochet Afro and lime green nails. Music of the month included "I Want You" by Luke James and "Waterfalls" by LVNDVN.

I was heavy on the music; it was the only thing getting me through August. "On Chill" by Wale and "All These Kisses" by Tammy Rivera. I kept myself motivated by wearing my hustle like your phone is on one percent T-shirt and keeping my perfect head tie wrapped on my head with my Janet Jackson Rhythm-Nation earrings. I drove to see friends who invited me out no matter how far the distance.

Things got so tight that I had to break down and put an ad out to rent rooms. I put my son and myself in one room and rented the other two bedrooms to cover the mortgage, leaving me to worry only about the utilities. This caused a bit of outrage from my siblings; I had to ignore that because they could not help financially.

I cut about three inches off of my hair and got a sharp bob in an effort to redefine and realign myself. The highlight of this time was a friend who took a liking to Issa offered to take him to various themed parks and events. Because of this, Issa experienced a lot of joy during this time, and I don't believe he noticed that I was having a hard time. He loved having extra people in the house. One of the tenants had a son who was a little younger than him, and they played on the weekends. To him, it was fun to have a playmate at home.

Some of my proudest work took place in August. I volunteered for an initiative called Class is in Session in Alexandria, VA. I donated hair services to children. Once the children's hair was done, they attended STEM, financial management, and dancing classes. At the end of the event, children were given book bags and supplies for the first day of school.

My son participated in the program while I volunteered. He was adored by the coordinator and told me all about his adventures that day on the ride home.

I took some risks with my hairstyles and outings. I wore one of the ugliest wigs known to man to a concert. The wig was so big! I love big hair, but the part was a mess. My friend couldn't make it to an R&B concert and offered me the tickets he had for his girlfriend and himself. I called a friend and asked him if he wanted to go, and he said sure, but he was acting super weird the entire night. I suspect he thought I was trying to hit on him because most of the concert was love songs. Maybe it was the wig. I really didn't know what I was getting into; I was just excited to go out. I hadn't been to a concert in a while. I didn't want to make it more awkward by asking him what was wrong, but made a note to self that something was up with him. I saw Ashanti perform that night, and that was the highlight of the evening.

August is for Me 2019

When my birthday came around, I had no plans because I had no money. My friend called me and said, "Get ready; I'm coming to pick you up."

I scurried to find two or three fabulous fits because she is the party girl, and I knew we wouldn't just go to one place. We went to dinner at an all-you-can-eat dining experience, and I loved it. The following day, we went to a nightclub during the dining hours and enjoyed two things we love—food and dance. This was a midweek celebration that I will never forget because it was just her and me. The timing was impeccable, taking place when I wasn't in the position to be dining out. Her full red-carpet treatment and hospitality made me forget about my hardship for two days. I wore a black glittery dress with feathers on the bottom and fiery red crinkle hair on day one. I wore a black and gold sequinned dress with a 54-inch body wave wig on day two. Serving I am sexy; I'm not depressed; I'm not lonely; I'm not impoverished.

This year had so much commotion and invites that not having sex wasn't difficult at all. What was tough was not being hugged or held. It is a feeling that provides comfort in despair, and besides the greeting from friends and family, it just wasn't there. Also, falling asleep at night was easy on the days that I was exhausted and tougher on the days I felt emotional about my grief, finances, and lack of support in raising my son.

CHAPTER 2

SEPTEMBER 2019

IN THE NICK OF TIME

(ONE YEAR)

It was my mom's one-year anniversary, and I didn't know what to expect. It was a very quiet day with minimal phone calls. That experience took me back to 2018. The times I assumed would be reflective, communal, or uplifting, there was silence. Toward the end of the day, I spoke with my Aunt Roxy and that was it. I did not like that feeling and told myself that I would make plans for her anniversary in the future.

Grandma's Birthday 2019

Before the loss of my mom, September belonged to Marian Hopkinson, my grandma, whose birthday is on the twenty-third. I usually found my way to New York to celebrate with her unless there were extenuating circumstances. It was time for the annual trip to Brownsville, Brooklyn, New York. During my visits, I spent most of the days speaking with my grandma. My son brought his guitar to play her songs, which she loved. I spent some time hanging out with my brother on my dad's side and my dad. I took pictures in front of Grandma's house as I did on every visit and walked the neighborhood with my son, telling him stories about where I fell off my bike and how far up the road I was allowed to ride my bike. I showed Issa Hopkinson Avenue (which has been renamed Thomas Boyland

Street) and told him stories about the old block parties and how things were so different in the early 1990s.

The sun was shining, and the heat of summer hadn't yet faded away. I wore my Genesis Barbershop T-shirt and shorts with my smart girl personality glasses and flick pics to my heart's content.

For Grandma's birthday, my aunt, whom I'm named after, came over with her husband and this completed our small bunch of the usual guests. My dad ordered Guyanese food and we listened to Guyanese folklore music. The night ended with reggae music. This annual gathering brought Grandma great joy.

In my October 2019 newsletter, I wrote about *Toy Story 4, The Secret Life of Pets 2, The Lion King, Spider-Man Far from Home, Hell's Kitchen, Dora,* and *the Lost City of Gold*. Five-Dollar Movie Tuesdays were something I took advantage of when my mom was sick. I looked forward to the movies because it was quiet and dark, and for two hours, I did not think about much. I continued going to the movies and eventually started writing reviews about the movies I watched. Movie watching increased from whenever I could make it to a mandatory Movie Tuesday requirement for my sanity.

In October, I went to my first Howard Homecoming event. I worked for Chase Bank on the experiential marketing team, preparing for the Howard Homecoming step show from start to finish. Every inch of the arena was dripping in Chase branding, from the wrapped doors to promotional T-shirts on every chair. I greeted Chase representatives in preferential seating and welcomed alumni chapters. It was great watching the main event. I was drawn to the art piece "The Divine Presence Creates a Divine Future" by Sydney James, which was painted throughout the day in my presence and completed just moments before guests arrived. Although I was there to help things run smoothly, it felt good to be fully aware of where I was and why the step show was important to others. I enjoyed it so much.

Growing up in a Caribbean-cultured household, one of the things my parents never taught me about was the Divine Nine (D9). Even though I participated and competed in my high school step team, I was not educated on the history of stepping, and I was completely ignorant that it was associated with fraternities and sororities. I knew that I loved doing it. It wasn't until my college years when my friend told me she was going to become a Sigma Gamma Rho, that I was introduced to Greek life. I went to her probate, and it was very exciting.

When I returned to my all-white private college, there was nothing to see. I didn't understand the magnitude or importance of D9 until I was much older. Many of my clients belonged to a sorority, and it was clear they were cut from a different cloth. They were all high achievers and self-starters. Imagine applying to colleges and being unaware of what a Historically Black College and University is (HBCU). It feels so embarrassing, but it shows that some guidance counselors and teachers are not telling students about the various types of education available. Ironically, my dad attended Tuskegee University, but I still hadn't made the connection.

I continued doing hair throughout the winter months while looking for ways to keep my child interested in education. In November, one of our most memorable trips was to two museums in DC—The Museum of Natural History, where Issa explored his love of dinosaurs, and The Museum of American History, where we had a chance to see the Batmobile, Captain America's shield and the old Wonder Woman costume. I was bedazzled by the first lady section; looking at their clothing inspired me to start saving pieces to wear to special events. In case I became famous, I wanted to make sure the curators had many outfits for my section in the museum.

On November 5, I celebrated my dad's sixty-first birthday by surprising him with an evening of live jazz. I learned of Paris Blues from watching *Paris Blues in Harlem.* The bar is tiny. The owner, Samuel Hargress II, was pleasant and extremely text-savvy. He bought my dad a splendid cake, and we enjoyed various songs throughout the evening. I am grateful I discovered it in time. The owner passed away on April 10, 2020. His historic club opened in 1969 and now it is closed indefinitely. Mr. Hargress was a civil rights activist who marched with Dr. Martin Luther King.

In late November, I was referred to do makeup for a short film, *Preparatory*, by one of my participants from the upcoming RAE2020. I was so excited at the opportunity. I thought one of the actors was so cute. His family was Guyanese too. We exchanged numbers right away. I quickly learned that he was collecting contacts of everyone on set. He had a girlfriend and was just being friendly. I looked at some of his photos online and noticed that they looked a tad flamboyant. I recommended him to my sister, but they never had a chance to connect for a shoot. As quickly as I put my eyes on him, I had to take them off. I invited him to do some creative work; he declined.

December tried to give me some sunshine, but the cloud of financial requirements would not let me be. My son had his first guitar recital and celebrated his first-year anniversary. He was all dressed up with his silver bow tie, and I was so proud. My uncle also allowed us to tag along at work, and Issa met Erykah Badu for the first time. He stood sidestage to listen to his favorite song of hers, "Hello," and spent most of the night in the band room, where everyone took turns giving him advice for his musical future. That was the best part of the month.

I revisited finishing the book I started in 2016 because now I knew how I wanted to end it. I also realized that I was running on a delusional loop and needed to get my story out to see if I could save anyone else from making the same mistakes.

I secured hair appointments by posting on social media, but it wasn't enough. I was styling women, men, kids. I even ventured into weaves. I don't think I was good at weaves because I never had a repeat customer. I was in big trouble by December 31. I was three months behind on the mortgage, and if I didn't pay by 2 p.m. on January 1, the bank would begin foreclosure on my mom's house. I tried everything I could legally think of, and I was still $700 short with one hour left until the deadline.

One of my Hair Therapy clients called me while I was pumping gas and watching the clock, completely stressed out.

She casually asked, "Hey girl, what are you doing?"

I somberly responded, "Trying to save my mom's house." She met me at the bank in fifteen minutes with cash in hand. The envelope had a note on it that read, "God loves you." I submitted the payment ten minutes before the deadline. That night, I could not speak. I was stunned and grateful. I almost let Mom's legacy slip through my fingers!

I thought in detail about every decision I had made in recent months. Did I spend Mom's reserve too fast? Did I underestimate how long it would take to get back on my feet? Life was hard and I could feel it. The way that better days came to be is truly unbelievable. The quickest recap was when my long-time Hair Therapy customer from back in 2013 referred her manager to me, who was looking for a stylist. I started doing his hair in December 2018. At the time, I was looking like a zombie and working to eat and survive.

In late 2019, I took the risk of letting him know I was in the market for a job, and he asked for my resume. He was floored by my experience and education. I interviewed shortly after and was presented with a contingent offer in October 2019. While waiting to hear back on the finalized terms of my employment, my life was falling apart. I was on the brink of losing my mom's house and wondering if I would end up like Justin Timberlake's mom, Rachel, in the movie *In Time*.

On January 2, 2020, the mortgage was paid, and I still felt like a character from *The Walking Dead*. I was especially annoyed because one of the tenants was laid off and stopped paying rent. I shook him down all of December, but he had nothing to give. In the third week of January, I received an offer and asked when I could start. I was so relieved by this positive news that I asked to come in the following Monday, which was Martin Luther King Day.

January 20 was a day I didn't believe in working; however, it was available for orientation and I took it. I wouldn't be at my actual job site; it was a day of formalities and onboarding paperwork. The same week the offer was given, my car was repossessed. December and January were the equivalent of being put through a meat grinder. My friend offered to send me an Uber for orientation. The ride was an hour each way. I can only imagine how much that Uber was, but thank goodness for friends who believe in you and have the resources to invest in you.

I didn't have a minute to spare or a romantic thought in January. I was running for everything I wanted and everything I needed. The first few weeks of work were rough. I had to get up at 5 a.m. to get there in time for 7 a.m. I didn't have anyone to watch Issa, and I relied on an iPad to call him to help him through the get-ready process and remind him when it was time to walk to the bus stop. One time, he missed the bus, and a stranger called me to tell me she had seen Issa standing on the curb and was concerned. My heart sank to the ground, and I was sure that I was going to go to jail or he would be taken by child protective services after she reported me. She didn't report me and offered to keep an eye out for Issa in the mornings going forward. With the support of my dad and my first check, I got my car back.

As if life was not hectic enough, I continued with invites and production of my second RAE show. I've never filed a tax return so fast. The show was on February 29, and at the top of the month, I had no funding, but I had faith. In prior years, it hadn't cost more than $3,000. My refunds were usually $2,500, and I was going to find a way, even if I had to scale it down.

I even had a cousin bold enough to ask, "Does your son even have presents? Why are you spending so much on an event?" I hate it when anyone tries to talk to me about Issa, especially if I did not ask. Issa's basic needs were met, and there was no need to bring him into the questioning. I asked myself, *What is driving me?* Barely recovered from having financial hardship, *Why am I investing my return into an event that is not profitable?* My conscience told me *It needs to be done. Who else is doing it for the people you know? Who is recognizing them? If not you, then who?*

While riding the wave of inspiration, I coughed, and once I started, I could not stop. After one day of drinking NyQuil to make it through the workday, I had to break down and tell them I could not come in. My body started to hurt from head to toe, and

I became afraid. I went to the hospital, where they ran various tests but couldn't tell me what was wrong. They gave me some medicine that didn't work much and sent me home.

I made a will and wrote a letter to my family. I believed it was the end of my days, and I was so debilitated. My aunt wouldn't come; she said she could not afford to get sick. I was alone. I cried hard when I had the energy. I was mad. I finally got the job I needed to get life back on track, and now I was going to die alone—unloved with only my son to discover me. It crushed and cringed me. After five days of Wegman's deliveries and Issa taking care of himself, I woke up and my head wasn't spinning. I didn't feel cured, but I felt enough relief to think perhaps the Grim Reaper was going to choose another person.

As soon as I was able, my first stop was the bank to get my paperwork notarized. I returned to work and continued the Hair Therapy hustle. For Valentine's Day, I attempted to plan a Galentine's to reduce the pinch of this commercialized lover's day. My cousin came down from New York, and the weekend plans were to host my annual makeup class, attend another friend's birthday dinner, and go to the movies to see *The Photograph*.

I sponsored my third makeup workshop on February 15. After weeks of promoting the two classes, one in the morning and one in the afternoon, one of the instructors canceled the night before, stating her boyfriend had made plans she didn't know about. I was so relieved that I booked two artists. I updated the info on my site to reflect one class and immediately unfollowed her. The class went well, we had a decent turnout, and the instructor was informative. I hosted it at Genesis Barbershop, and the set-up for each lady at the individual barber station was super cute.

I am the queen of placing myself at the center of complex situations. Classic Man was at the birthday dinner. It wasn't a complete shock because he is my friend's family member but it was not confirmed he would attend. I had not seen him in person in a while. My ears were hot; I thought I would overheat and pass out. He had a haircut and looked very classic. I was wearing my mom's ring. He asked if I was engaged, I asked if he was married, and he fell silent. I literally wanted to sit on his lap, but in the name of decorum, I ate my soup. I thought about dinner the whole ride home.

The next day, the girls who said they were interested in the movie all flaked, and it ended up just being my cousin and me. To make matters worse, I took too long to buy tickets while waiting for others, and we ended up in the first row! The movie was good, but the neck-breaking angle, not so much.

RAE2020

Shortly after Valentine's weekend, my tax refund came in, and I had seven days to hire a chef and DJ and secure a venue. Chef Rob, who attended the first RAE as a guest, agreed to cater, and Codie, a current participant, gave me a great deal on using his commercial space.

The most amazingly disastrous thing was that one of the men I approached to participate rejected the offer but referred me to a point of contact from Moet. They agreed to sponsor the event. There was an error made by a staff member who did not ship on time, and instead of getting eight cases, we received four cases from an emergency carrier.

One of my participants was given a surprise trip by his wife and could not attend. Another dropped out, and I replaced him with Issa, who stole the show. The crowd loved his interview. We partied like it was 1999, with no idea what was in store for us.

Anyone who avoided the news hoping for the best was slapped in the face during March. In addition to circulating images of coffins and videos of infected celebrities, toilet paper flew off the shelves. The phrase "social distancing" was coined and popularized. Work-from-home tests were rolled out by various companies. Mall workers were laid off, and the announcement was made that Virginia public schools would be closed for the rest of the year.

On the day of the school closure announcement, a single tear rolled down my face. My first thoughts were: OMG. How bad is this shit?! If they don't care about education anymore, we are probably all about to die! Then I thought, my son finally has a teacher I loved and had developed a great communication system with. How am I supposed to be a provider and a homeschool teacher? My shoulder hurt, and my back felt like I was carrying something heavy.

Notifying my son that he would not return to school was the hardest thing I had to do. He cried immediately. He was disheartened that he did not have a chance to say goodbye to his friends.

Luckily, with the help of FaceTime, I helped him connect with his teacher the next day. She held two weekly Zoom meetings, one on Monday and one on Friday, where he could interact with classmates. After securing some numbers, he FaceTimed with his favorite classmates on the weekends. Although nothing compared to in-person interactions, I saw a significant rise in my son's spirit.

After some deliberation, I decided that it was important for him to continue music lessons. Initially, we skipped one week due to the acute stress the sudden change had on both of us. The following week, we made up the session, meeting on Monday and Thursday. The biggest benefit of online music lessons was the reduction in price—guitar lessons cost $30 less a month.

I stopped seeing clients in March, about two weeks before barbershops and salons officially closed. It was difficult to turn down my clients' requests with no definitive answer of when I would be available again. Although I did their hair at home and did not see as many people as I used to in the shop, I developed a great bond with the clients I had. They are like my family, and it was like saying no to my brothers, sisters, aunties, and Grandma. I made quarantine beauty videos documenting how I was staying presentable during the pandemic with no professional assistance. I was in my two-strand Marley twist era. I had black roots and royal blue ends. It was tiring to put extensions in your own hair, and I almost never finished the middle of my head.

Work changed from a hybrid schedule to fully remote Monday through Friday. I didn't have a significant other to be quarantined with; it was just Issa and me. I received some "Are you OK?" texts, which did nothing to combat the fear of the world's fate.

April is for Issa 2020

On Issa's birthday (April 5), we started the morning early with a fresh loc retwist and took pictures around the corner from the house. For the first time, he had a cinnamon roll instead of a cupcake for his birthday song. The iPhone I ordered after his missing the bus incident arrived. It was not as purposeful as intended now that we were both stuck in the house, but he was so excited to have his very own phone.

In May, I watched so much TV and made many videos. *The Last Dance* (ESPN), *For Life* (ABC), *Little Fires Everywhere*

(Hulu), *Ozark* (Netflix), *Becoming* (Netflix). I could never get enough of Michael Jordan. I've heard people say many different things about him, and it falls on deaf ears when they talk to me. I think he is amazing. The grit. From watching him on games as a kid, to the "Be Like Mike" commercial and watching him tell his own story. The impact on basketball is undeniable, but beyond basketball, it's a lesson in discipline. When I see the number 23, I think get up and work on your skill every day. I can't play a lick of basketball, but I'll be purchasing Jordan's until I'm six feet under. One of my biggest fears is looking like one of those adults that don't know when it is time to let go of the clothes they wore in high school. Most of my Jordan purchases are for Issa. I had him watch the documentary with me so he could understand more about why all the kids in school look like clones and wear those shoes and how all the hoopla over Jordan's began.

June arrived. School was out and instead of feeling relief about summer break, a different kind of stress was mounting. Every time I woke up, I was instantly disappointed that life was not a dream. I live in the U.S., where the KKK supported the president. Where, since slavery ended, Black men have been criminalized to exploit the portion of the revised thirteen Amendment that made prisoners slaves. Do I actually live in a time when there are more people in jail than there were in "slavery?" Where the land that makes up five percent of the world's population is the home of twenty-five percent of the world's prisoners!

The racial issues are not new and have been compounding my entire life. I had never felt stress to the point of sleep deprivation until I realized that my son would grow up to be a target and viewed as a walking threat if things in the U.S. do not change for the better. My therapist concluded that my worries for Issa's future, coupled with hysteria caused by the coronavirus, Black men being killed and converted to hashtags every month, mistreatment of protesters streaming nonstop on Facebook, and the murder of George Floyd and mounting lynching cases to be the complete cause of acute stress. Now, I think I can diagnose all Black moms in America with the same case of "WTF" that I have.

Issa learned of slavery in-depth when I took him to the African American Museum last year. I told him the entire building was dedicated to Black History, and he responded, "I'm Black?!" and everyone looked at me. This was truly an example that children are born a blank slate. Issa was angry to see and learn more of this history. The only thing that calmed his spirit was seeing Frederick Douglas and Lincoln, who he learned "freed" the slaves in school. He also coped by thinking of slavery and racism as a thing of the past. He spoke of the injustice and referenced the chains he saw for weeks.

I deliberated for days before I told him about what was happening in the world. Remembering how the discussion of slavery surprised and saddened him, I used news reports and some of my own words to tell Issa what happened to George Floyd. He was angry, and his first response was, "I want to beat the police with a stick." On that particular night, DC was on fire. When I showed Issa the picture, he said, "We are getting our payback, Mom." I said, "We are going to sleep, and we will figure out what we can do to help the cause when we wake up." I did take him to DC to see where protesters were marching. By this time, most of the crowd had died down because the community had been out there for weeks.

My discomfort regarding the state of America led to more Black History research, specifically concerning hair. I shared my findings with my readers about how cornrows were used to smuggle rice from Africa to the Caribbean and the US and recommended the book *Black Rice* by Judith Carney. The book tells a story of how hair played a major part in the cultivation of agriculture in America. I shared my newfound knowledge on the Tignon laws created for Black women to cover their hair so white men wouldn't be attracted to women of color and how Black women turned punishment into a fashion statement. Although reading about these stories made me so upset, my takeaway was:

- Always be resilient
- Black women must be unique and exquisite if such extreme measures were taken to hide their hair.

I felt proud every time I wore my natural hair out or tied up and extra cool to have a hair tie line. Very proud of Black women's creativity, I sported black and purple hair. Black Marley twists at the root and lilac loose hair at the bottom. I was flattered when I shared the images, and one of the comments said I looked "majestic." You don't hear that every day.

In an effort to get away on a budget and explore the great outdoors, I planned a one-day adventure to the Natural Bridge, Roaring Run, and Falling Springs. The Natural Bridge is three hours from my house. This automatically added six hours to the trip. Three hours to get the starting point and start the loop. The Lace Falls at the Natural Bridge was smaller than expected; the Bridge itself, which took millions of years to form, was a wonder. The very well-paved trail was a relaxing walk, but Lace Falls at the end of that trail was underwhelming. Issa pointed out all the little tadpoles.

Roaring Run was tough to find, and the GPS had me rolling in circles. Falling Springs was gushing out of a rock, and I saw it from the corner of my eye as I drove down the street.

It was a zero-hike waterfall. It was once allowed to walk to the bottom, but it has been fenced off due to multiple people injuring themselves. I wish Covington weren't five hours away. I could visit more often. After all that driving, I was ready to stop at the esteemed Omni Homestead Resort. The restaurant I wanted to visit was closed, so I ordered a veggie burger from another restaurant on the grounds. We took a few pics and geared up for the ride home.

The next day, I was in terrible pain. I went to the doctor, who referred me to a gastroenterologist. She gave me a medicine that tasted like chalk and killed all the bacteria in my body. Not to be dramatic, but I think I was poisoned at the resort. I saw more Confederate flags on my way to these falls than I have seen driving across the entire country. I was curled in a ball for most of July and wondered if I'd make it to my birthday. I had been in bed for weeks, and I wasn't feeling better.

August is for Me 2020

August started with a bang. A photo that was taken of me in 2015 went viral, being posted and reposted on various pages. I picked up a few head tie sales because of it. The show, *The Chi*, was the talk of the town. I was also immensely invested in *P-Valley*. Andre reminded me of someone I knew. When I wasn't power washing a fence or buying solar lights, I was at a friend's baby shower or birthday party. There were no dull moments; there were many things to do.

My dad made a surprise visit (possibly a wellness check) on the twenty-seventh, and I could not have been happier! It was time to celebrate surviving an adventurous solar return on August 28, 2020. My month was here!! I was beginning to glow. My bills were paid; I had a weekend of fun planned. We did a paint and sip at home. I had a spa day at the Salamander

Resort in Middleburg, Virginia. We had lunch, massages, and waded in the pool. I capped off the festivities with a private chef-catered dinner at home with two close friends. A few people asked me if it was a milestone, insinuating it was a bit much for an odd number like thirty-seven. I paid them no mind. I felt good to celebrate living. My friends got me the most thoughtful gifts and cards. I felt so special.

CHAPTER 3

SEPTEMBER 2020

CHASING WATERFALLS

(TWO YEARS)

After the birthday high wore off, Mom's second anniversary was a day away. This time, I had plans, and I took September 2 off. Issa and I started the day at Quantico Park, where my mom saw her final sunset. We looked at the water and took a few pictures, but we both felt emotional and didn't stay as long as I had hoped.

Next, we visited a garden I learned about while doing online searches for peaceful places in Virginia. Our road trip began heading to Richmond to visit the Lewis Ginter Botanical Garden for the first time. I heard sniffles in the back seat and asked Issa if he was OK. He said he was, but I knew he was sad.

I said, "It is OK to cry, Issa." He didn't bawl, only silent tears. My heart felt heavy, and I wanted to pull over that instant, but I kept on driving with a bleeding heart. It felt like a razor nicked my heart. Each breath hurt as I held back the tears.

The grounds at the Botanical Gardens were charming and colorful. There was a lot of open space to explore. It had sculptures and cobblestone walkways. It reminded me of how I imagined the secret garden would look when I read the book some years ago. I brought my mom's huge 23x18 picture with us so we could take pictures with it. A passerby who happened to be a photographer took the best picture for us. Issa was holding one corner, and I was holding the other. It felt good to be there.

My mom was constantly cleaning the yard. She didn't plant many colorful flowers. One rose bush with pink flowers and one bush that blossomed with white flowers. Everything else was green. I thought about how much Issa had grown since my mom was gone and how much my pantsuit sleeveless jumper looked like an outfit she would be proud of. I felt the sunshine and listened to the water fountains. I was reassured that it was a great decision to visit the gardens.

Cascades Falls

From Richmond, we headed to Blacksburg to see Cascades Falls. The sun was about to set when we arrived at the park. I asked one of the hikers how long it took to walk the trail; they said it took about an hour and didn't recommend that we start so late. We could get stuck in the forest in the dark. We checked into a nearby hotel as we had driven too far not to see it. Issa was so pumped to stay some place new. We both felt relaxed and comfortable in our shower robes and had a much-needed night of rest.

First thing in the morning, I attempted to log into my work computer, but the welcome screen read "access revoked." Revoked!!! That sounded bad. I called IT, and the tech tried to help me. He said that nothing on his end was working, and I may want to request a new access card. I called the manager to let him know I didn't have access and was worried because of the revoked message. He told me not to worry and take the day off.

The Cascades Falls hike was rough and not for kids or rookie hikers. The feeling of getting to it was rewarding. When we were halfway there, Issa complained that his feet hurt. When a passing hiker said it was another mile, I wanted to jump off the trail and end it all. Instead, I told Issa we would take our time and get there eventually, and we did. It was at that moment that I realized we were on a four-mile voyage—two miles in and two miles back.

When we arrived, there were people in the water. I couldn't imagine getting wet and being damp on the way back to the car. We took selfies and sat on a big rock taking in the scenery. I was still thinking about my revoked access card. We had to take little steps to get back to the car as Issa was tired. It took hours, but I could not carry him. I wanted to shoot a flare gun and get rescued by a helicopter. According to CNN's list of the best waterfalls across the U.S., only one is in Virginia: Cascades Falls, listed at number seven. I am happy to have made it there, but I am not going back. I vowed to read all the park details and look at the miles it takes to get to the main attraction in the future.

Once I returned home, I scheduled a meeting to get a new card. When I went in, they confiscated my computer and told me I was off the contract. The manager had no idea what was going on or why. I received a call on September 11, a date of national tragedy, as well as the day my mom was cremated. I was told it was discovered that I was unfit for a cleared position. The person who deactivated me left the agency, so the proper channels of notification were not followed. All I could do was blink. She went on to say they had a program called Family First, which I was placed in. I would be paid for two weeks while they try to put me in another position. I had one interview for the communications department.

The interviewer asked me if I was interested in communications why was my recent position in IT. I wanted to say, "Bitch because I need money. I have a fucking Master's in Communications. Are you questioning my love for it? What the fuck kind of dumb-ass question is that?"

Instead, I said, "The IT opportunity arose from a closely developed business relationship, and I decided to take it. I am currently looking for a position that fits my area of expertise." I knew she was not going to hire me, and that is a terrible feeling when you are in a tough spot. On the twenty-eighth, my company cut a check, and that was it. I was an employee nowhere again!!

School was in full effect, and Issa was in third grade with his favorite teacher, Ms. Bentley. He met Miss Bentley in second grade when she was a substitute, and she took a liking to him. She was his teacher, but not in person. My new full-time job was supporting Issa through online learning. I had already called my dad crying once about how it was too distracting to have Issa home trying to learn while I was at work. I was not asking for my job to be removed. I thought, *Maybe I need to be careful about how I complain*.

The IT guy who had tried to help me found me on LinkedIn. I noticed right away and said, "Hey, I am not on LinkedIn often; I am on IG." We became IG friends and met up shortly after that. He was cute and tall. He was also asleep. We were chatting and watching a movie, and he was asleep. I hate when people fall asleep in movies, even at home. Ugh. I was certainly tripping because hanging out at home for a first hangout never worked out well for any woman ever. He continued to be a spotty texter and worked my nerves. I spent the rest of September taking hair appointments while worrying about being unemployed. I was not able to visit Grandma for her birthday due to my crisis. I also prepared to host a virtual book club meet-up with my mentor.

Book Club

The book club started as a virtual brunch. Feeling a bit blue about the impossibility of a face-to-face 2020 Brunch Tour, I took a shot at having a virtual brunch on May 31. It was great; we spoke about the current state of the world, race relations, safety, stress, and the importance of therapy. Guest appearances were made by Dr. Groff, reverend and educator, and Ms. Jackson, a licensed therapist. We set a date to meet again on Juneteenth (June 19). During the Juneteenth meet-up, my sister, NikkRich (a professional photographer), was on the call. She spoke about how the artificial urgency to work with Black people has been created in the Hollywood photography industry and how it has affected her choices of who to work with.

Following the trend of meeting on holidays, the July 4 call was more of a welfare check-in. The discussion was centered around questions such as, Did anyone give in to celebrating July 4? If yes, why? How do we feel about white people asking us if we are OK? How do we effectively respond to what is going on? After much private deliberation with my peers, Dr. Miles Davis joined the call to offer a few words of perspective. Instantly, we all became enrolled in an unofficial class of history and critical thinking.

Dr. Davis was the sitting president of Linfield University in Oregon. He challenged us to start with ourselves—protect our family, check on our neighbors, which strengthens the community, join causes that support our beliefs, and vote. He also recommended that we read the book, *The Mis-Education of the Negro,* by Carter G. Woodson and promised to join the next call if the group completed the book.

I am not much of a reader, and I pushed through the assignment by listening to the audio version on Kindle to complete the book by the due date of September 9. Wednesday, September 9, 2020, was my first time using a book as a reference to address my modern-day concerns with my peers. It was an engaging and positive experience. Dr. Davis's next suggested read was *The Souls of Black Folk* by W.E.B DuBois. The recommendation was warmly received by the group. The next discussion was set for October 31.

My first kiss popped back into my life through Facebook. We had a short chat, and it was a nightmare. He went on about how former President Obama didn't do anything for Black people. He opposed every comment I made, and it seemed that he was a passionate Republican, but he also refused to admit it. I invited him to the October virtual book club discussion, and he got on my nerves there too. Dr. Davis always remained calm and answered most of his comments with historical context. Something I was not able to do. All I know is he was getting on my fucking nerves.

He called me after the meet-up and continued to troll more while making some sexual advances. He told me I was almost perfect; I was just misguided. I told him to suck my dick. He was insanely offended, and we both started cursing at the top of our lungs. I wish I could slam the phone, but I had to settle for hitting the end button. He was still handsome and well-dressed. He was a CPA, and he would tell anyone who would listen how high his credit score was. He even posted a screenshot of it. Ugh, he was so obnoxious. I used to love seeing pics of his cute son on social media, but I was sure I wanted to disconnect all ties with him. We were too incompatible even for friendship.

I styled and ate my way through October. I made some really cool creative visuals. I used jackets and converted them into head ties. BCBG Max Azria liked my post, which was encouraging. I worked on the promo videos for my book with my trusted photographer, Kevin, which was always a pleasure. I knew I wanted the cover to be sexy, and I wanted to release some mini commercials. I stayed active, but I still felt my self-esteem going lower and lower as the days went by. It felt like the carpet was ripped from under me, and I couldn't shake it. My productivity was going down.

The men in my daily life were paid to be there. I had a Black contractor, handyman, and chef. I called them when I needed help with things, mainly on Saturdays. They helped with tiling in the kitchen and cleaning the shed, which was full of crickets that scared me to death. I purchased a pan stir-fry rice from time to time. The pan was huge and afforded me a two-day break from cooking. I spent an enormous amount of my days cooking. I made walnut banana pancakes, chocolate chip pancakes with grilled bananas, sweet potato pies, sixteen-bean soup, homemade pizza with carrots and broccoli seasoned in garlic, yellow peppers, extra virgin olive oil, and topped with sesame seeds. I mastered vegan spaghetti and found the perfect recipe for vegan s'mores. Cooking was cost-effective and delicious, yet sometimes I needed a break.

Winter

I had been excited to use this winter break to catch up on shows. The show that blew me away was *Ramy*. I was a bit late to the party since season one of this show aired April 19, 2019. I eased into the show with no expectations. I identify most with Ramy's struggle to be true to his faith and still wanting to indulge in everything! Low-key Ramy was a POS because he repeatedly made terrible decisions and hurt others. The language in the show is wild. Several groups were represented in this series—first-generation Egyptians, African American Muslims, disabled persons, white males, and veterans. Pressures represented in the series include societal, religious, marital, and sexual. Issues represented double standards, porn, incest, and racism. My favorite character in the show is Sheikh Malik, played by Mahershala Ali. The first time I heard him pray, I was touched.

Jingle Jangle, *Soul,* and *Ma Rainey's Black Bottom* were also on my watch list. It was hard to accept the loss of Chadwick Boseman, and I was determined to support the last film he was featured in. I hated it when he died fictitiously in *Avengers: Endgame* and was broken-hearted when he died in real life. I got lost in my movies and shows and considered myself the local version of Rotten Tomatoes, even taking extra steps to rate the movies.

Another winter, another mortgage crisis. The ends were not meeting, unemployment ended, and I hadn't found a new job yet. My therapist told me about a program called EHAP, which was a crisis program for people having trouble paying their mortgage. It was a lengthy application, and they asked for many supporting documents. I was pretty nervous when they asked why my name was not on the mortgage. I needed the money, and I wasn't sure if telling the truth was going to disqualify me. She called me and said, in an effort to be sensitive, she would like to know if my mom was alive. I told her no.

She said, "I am so sorry. Please provide the death certificate, and we will continue to process your case." On December 14, she emailed that I was approved for six months of mortgage payments. I was so stunned. Sometimes, when things are bad, I think, What did I do to deserve this? At that moment, I thought about how blessed I was to have the therapist and case worker I was assigned. This was a special kind of therapy—the kind that helps with my mind and my housing. The approval stamped a lesson I learned a while ago and continue to practice. All great changes start with an application.

The New Year came with PTSD. Issa's paternal grandma was diagnosed with cancer and did not share the news until she was near the end of life. On January 9, we visited her, and her arm was swollen. Issa's dad, Issa's sister, and his sister's mom were there. We sat in the living room, and Grandma asked the kids the usual things: how they were doing in school and if they were being good. I was perturbed that I was experiencing another cancer-related loss and wished they had more time. Grandma's sister commented that she had not been speaking much, and the kids gave her a spark and burst of energy. Issa's grandma passed away days later.

It was inauguration time, and the series of events over the past four years, compounded by the visible rage expressed during the past few weeks, made the moment even sweeter. Time stood still today. During the wake of destruction, hatred, and difference of opinion, a significant number of Black women organized how they wanted to be seen and heard through what has become known as the "fight for democracy." Madam Vice President stepped into her new role wearing Black designers Christopher John Rogers and Sergio Hudson. I never thought I would see the day in America. I really could not believe my eyes.

At the top of February, I was in the final editing stages of *Beautiful Reject: Seven Years of Delusional Dating,* and I began to get nervous. I found a great copy editor because growing up, I received lots of dings on my papers for spelling errors and grammar, and I feared my book would have too many errors if it wasn't edited. I was falling asleep listening to videos on YouTube about how to self-publish. I made a mock version of the cover on my phone, and I shopped for someone on Upwork to format the cover and the book. I was learning as I was going and hoped to reach my deadline and desired release date of February 14. On the thirteenth, I waited until midnight to upload my stuff and waited impatiently for it to get approved. I was nervous. What if people thought the book was stupid? Did I add enough research to the book?

I also wasn't in the best state of mind as I had made a huge declaration of goodbye to Classic Man a few days prior. I will say that social media will give you images your heart can't handle. He was moving on with his life, and I was sick of being his fucking pen pal. This added to my nerves. He is an avid reader. What will he think of the things I wrote about him? Will anyone in my life "Best Man" me or treat me like Wendy Williams? Will anyone read it at all?

There was a huge relief once everything was published. I felt so proud. I went from talking about it and giving up on it to finally completing it. My friend pointed out that there was no resolution for one of the characters, Mr. Green Eyes. I honestly did not notice. My fingers were smoking while writing about Classic Man because I wrote some sections of the book out of order, and I think my brain was fried after that.

I probably should give her a copy of this book before sending it to print. For the ones just dying to know, Mr. Green Eyes dated my college boyfriend's older sister after dating me. He had a baby with her. I almost choked when I saw their picture on Facebook. I really didn't see that coming. That was the worst version of "It's a small world after all." He was literally living in my past, and I could never rejoin that family. Some men from my past found sections about themselves and reached out. No one yelled at me. They said things like, "Page 28 sounds familiar." A piece of me wondered, *did you read the whole thing or were you just looking for yourself?*

Bridgerton had the people walking around saying, "Your Grace" as a greeting. I didn't read the books; I didn't know what to expect from the show. I enjoyed seeing the outfits, the visualization of Black royalty, and the complex relationship between the Duke of Hastings and Daphne Bridgerton, the princess. It was so romantic and sexy. Of everything I watched that month, it was the most captivating. It had me dreaming that someone would whisper sweet nothings in my ears. I swirled around from February to March. This time felt different than the others. I had to get away from the cycle that I was in. How can I be such an idiot and keep breaking my own heart over and over again? I was jealous that the people of my past were making families and going on vacations while I was home alone watching movies. Do I not deserve that happy ending? Why can't I have what I want? The options were breadcrumbs and nothing. I desired neither. I wanted it all. Except for a dog. I have never had a desire to have a dog.

Judas & the Black Messiah and *The United States vs. Billie Holiday* were small band-aids for my big wounds. The spirit of escapism was upon me. The sound of water is supposed to be healing, so I planned a three-day escape for us. Issa was approaching age nine and about to celebrate his second birthday during the pandemic. Issa was 100 percent virtual; he attended school, doctor appointments, and guitar lessons online. His meltdowns were increasing, which reminded me of the side effects of solitary confinement I learned about.

Triple Falls, Looking Glass, Dry Falls

Since Issa and I have seen all of Virginia's notable waterfalls, including the best-voted Falling Spring Falls, I started researching waterfalls in neighboring states. North Carolina recently piqued my interest because it is home to over 250 waterfalls and houses three amazing things. First, the only waterfall I came across that you can walk behind is Dry Falls in Highlands. Second, one of the best vegan restaurants in the country, according to *The Food_Network*, Plant in Asheville. Third, information about Black Wall Street.

Learning lessons from the first **waterfall** tour in Virginia, I triple-checked the addresses. I was devastated to learn that Dry Falls was the furthest waterfall from my home. It was basically falling out of North Carolina and a whopping eight hours away if I drove there straight. I knew I wanted to see three falls minimum. I searched for drive-by falls and falls with short hikes. I added Looking Glass, known for being easily accessible, and High Falls, noted for its appearance in *The Hunger Games*.

With the waterfalls toward the end of North Carolina and Plant hours away from the falls, I decided to create a loop so I didn't miss out on all North Carolina had to offer. It took hours of Google Maps to find points of interest, vegan carry-outs, and operation times. I used some backward math to calculate the necessary departure times. I timed everything based on arriving at the opening time for each carry-out, and I was successfully the first customer for each carry-out.

I saw every planned point of interest. In Dupont State Park, I switched out High Falls for Triple Falls. High Falls had a trail that led to another trail. Once we completed the first trail, we were greeted by two signs for High Falls Loop and didn't know which one to take. The map was at the front of the park, and the internet on the phone wasn't working.

Issa immediately said, "No, Mommy, no."

Sometimes it is best to listen to the kids. We went to eat and recharge at Madison's in Old Edwards Inn before heading to Dry Falls. We were hungry and wet from getting rained on at Looking Glass, and the camera battery died! Having lunch first gave us time to recharge while visiting the historic, posh, and restored Inn.

Looking Glass is like the warmup to Dry Falls. Truly a baby version. It was easy to see from the roadside and not difficult to access the base of it. Dry Falls was my favorite waterfall experience to date. It was so powerful. No confusing trails, just a long set of steps leading straight to the natural wonder. The water was so loud. When I stood underneath it, the feeling was exhilarating. What a refreshing perspective.

Asheville River Arts District had art on the walls that was so bold that we had to pull over. Apparently, the BBQ spot there is so good that former President Obama went to visit 12 Bones Smokehouse twice. There was no quick way to leave Asheville, so we didn't. We explored and found an art shop where the owner was a Batman and Marvel enthusiast, amongst other things. In Asheville, we also visited The Biltmore Estate, a tourist trap worth seeing. Getting to it is quite a production. It has a box office! It also has a trolley system. I had no interest in touring inside. I just needed my baby to see the biggest house in the US because he has an affinity for architecture.

My sole purpose for stopping in Greensboro was to show Issa the International Civil Rights Museum. It was informative and great to see the original stools where Greensboro Four pushed back on segregation and the 1960 sit-ins began. It was chilling to see a water fountain specifically for use by the "colored." We received local intel about Gateway Gardens, a cool garden/oasis created for kids. I delayed departing Greensboro to make sure Issa was able to visit. We were both a little sad when our adventure was over. The trip was a joy, and Gateway Gardens was a great ending. We left during the golden hour and took the cutest selfie, wearing matching NASA shirts. I learned while spending time with my son, and these adventures were so much fun. It felt like we were on our own reality TV show, and no one else existed.

April is for Issa 2021

All the waterfall fun was during spring break; for Issa's birthday, we did the usual. Hair styling first thing in the morning. Very cool Spider-Man shirt. We went to the playground and tried to fly the kite we bought at the Lewis Ginter Garden. We could barely get it off the ground. We ended the day with the family and friends on FaceTime, where I shared his annual birthday day video with all our latest adventures. I cried a million times making it.

When I wasn't chasing waterfalls, I was recreating spaces at home and going to see clients in person. In May, I converted Issa's room from the hot chocolate and whipped cream (brown and white) room he had when he came home from the hospital into a navy blue and white Spider-Man-themed room.

I updated my website and created a new online store with mugs, hoodies, and children's onesies. I was most proud of creating my second hair product, the Power Blend Hair Oil, with the help of Karen Saunders, creator of Karen Body Beautiful. I didn't sell many bottles. Ordering the product cost a thousand dollars, and I sold maybe twenty bottles. It was a little disappointing to have this great website and great product, and the only thing that made a profit was styling hair. I could not figure out how to break into e-commerce.

Issa and I went to New York to visit my dad and Grandpa Ron, my Mom's dad. He played music for his grandpa Ron. Grandpa was so surprised that we had taken the long ride out to Long Island to see him. Issa delivered red roses for his Aunty P, and she cried. She shared with me that back in the day, my mom would show up unannounced with red roses. She still had the dried petals in a jar. I realized that Issa was a joy to any grown-up. I wanted to share that love that only kids can give.

May was when I discovered Issa had video editing talent. He made a video for me for Mother's Day with images he found on the internet, and I was in tears. I was so surprised.

I also made it a goal to start working out in May. I took a friend up on an offer to learn Muay Tai and work out a bit. My friend nicknamed him SWG (savage with glasses). She deemed some of his actions to be surprising as she suspected he was holding back his true nature behind his glasses. When we started this journey, I was quickly reminded of how out of shape I was. I could barely keep up with him. When the workouts were over, we walked the trail, which was my favorite part of these meet-ups. We sometimes spoke on the phone about all kinds of things—current events, sports, and the past. I told him that I didn't really like unannounced FaceTime. Of course, he FaceTimed me, and that began the era of our regular FaceTimes. On Fridays, before we got off the phone, he would say, "What time tomorrow?" and that became our routine.

After a few weeks, I began to think there was hope for me to become fit after all. June came with many graduations and birthday invites, and I went to them all. Two of my Hair Therapy kids graduated high school, and one of my Hair Therapy ladies received her Master's. One of my friends had a fabulous fiftieth on Juneteenth. I was a part of a surprise party for another friend who survived breast cancer. Sadly, in June, one of my cousins died from COVID-19. She was close with my dad, and he came to Maryland for her funeral. She was the first person that I knew who died from the virus.

Dr. Groff recommended Issa for a virtual summer camp with Auburn University. The camp was two weeks, and I made the biggest deal about it like he was going away to college forever. I loved that the program was led by faculty at the

University. It wasn't a camp run in a university space by students and aspiring teachers; instead, it was run by PhD holders and curriculum creators.

I was sharing every turn of information with my Hair Therapy newsletter readers, and they gave me encouraging words about my articles and recommendations. I think I even inspired my dad—the only reader who clicks every link. My dad called one sunny afternoon and said he wanted to take a road trip to California! I made the journey twice before. Once, in 2006, when I thought I would become a print model after college, and in 2015, when I helped my sister move. I drove there with her and flew back alone. This would be my first time with my dad and son, and I was down for the challenge and adventure.

I traveled and visited twenty-five states (Maryland, Delaware, New Jersey, New York, Pennsylvania, Ohio, Michigan, Indiana, Illinois, Minnesota, Wisconsin, Wyoming, South Dakota, Utah, Nevada, California, Arizona, New Mexico, Texas, Louisiana, Mississippi, Alabama, Georgia, and Tennessee). I ate a lot of food and saw many things.

When we visited the Ohio Rock and Roll Hall of Fame, Prince Issa was excited to see Michael Jackson's outfits and elated that Jimi Hendrix's guitar looked just like his replica. The scariest routes I drove at night were in Wyoming; no lights and countless deer. Detroit, Michigan, was the most heartbreaking living conditions and dangerous environment I visited. Minnesota, the home of Prince and George Floyd, forced me to reflect and feel deeply for Black men in the nation. The best landscape I saw was in Utah.

The coldest city and foggiest city was San Francisco. San Francisco had the biggest pride flag I have ever seen. The most relaxing feeling was early mornings listening to the Pacific

Ocean on Bruce Beach in California. The best food I ever tasted was in New Orleans at GW Fins. The Kimpton Hotel there was lovely. Many of the streets in the neighborhoods of New Orleans were flooded, and cars were almost one-quarter submerged. The Welcome to Virginia sign on the Tennessee border was worth a picture even if it is home because that particular sign is five hours away from Northern Virginia, and I don't see it often.

My dad and I took turns speeding across the country; we spoke about so many things. He told me about some of his dating stories. That is how I knew I was officially grown up. I told him that I had a not-so-great experience. He said, "Daughter, I am learning that as much as you speak, there is a lot you don't tell me, and I'm sorry you went through that."

I always hesitated to tell my dad about the sexual abuse because he did a great job taking care of me. No sleepovers ever. I have never been touched or molested by anyone. He protected me from everything. I felt like it would disappoint him that I couldn't protect myself. I even thought he would think I threw all his efforts away with my poor decisions in men. Ultimately, I was projecting and ashamed. I was ashamed that the experience happened and my response to it.

When we returned home, I thought about the trip for weeks and how incredible the timing was that I was an entrepreneur, Issa was out of school, and Dad was available. The way the trip started was crazy—on my way to get my dad, I hit a pothole going over a bridge. I took the nearest exit and had to pull over on the side of the highway because I couldn't make it any further.

My dad kept saying, "How did you end up in the Bronx if you were on the way to Brooklyn?" I found Jerome's 24-hour car service. They put the car on the flatbed with Issa and I still inside the car! Is that even legal? I was looking out the window in shock. I had a new tire $180 later and proceeded to pick up my dad. When I pulled up, my dad said, "You are unstoppable and determined." I smiled. I like starting my long road trips late at night; this debacle took place between 2 a.m. and 3 a.m. I had every minute of our ten days planned out, and I wouldn't let a tire derail us from staying on track.

It was time to switch gears into something serious. I was scheduled for surgery July 27, 2021, after complaining to my doctor about the lumps in the extra tissue under my armpits. I've always had extra breast tissue under both of my armpits. One was getting bigger than the other, and when I was on my cycle, it felt like a pebble was in the middle of each armpit. I complained in the past and was told it was nothing. This time, I had a Black female doctor who referred me to a specialist. He took a sonogram and said, "I can take it out next week. I can only do one side." He said if he requested to do both sides, insurance would deny the claim and say it was cosmetic surgery. I don't know if I should have pushed for both or gone back soon after to do the left side.

Once he removed the tissue from the right and tested the cyst, it came back benign with no sign of cancer. He said it was hormonal, and if I had more kids, it was a possibility it could come back. My sister helped with the drain that he put in; blood made my knees weak, and a little cup of blood needed to be emptied.

I issued a statement through my newsletter that I was stepping away from styling hair permanently and transitioning into e-commerce. Although I could return to styling after recovery, I really did not want to do it anymore. The standing, the schlepping, the schedule—it was all getting to me. The prime time for styling was Saturday. I had been giving up Saturdays for years and wanted them back. My vision was for my products to sell like the Mielle organics products I used.

August is for Me 2021

After three weeks of recovery at home, I was ready just in time to step out for another year of birthday celebration activities. This year, I had black soft locs, cheetah stiletto nails, and makeup by my talented younger cousin. I looked good! I started the tradition of making time to take Issa to dinner. I had the idea to go on the twenty-seventh, which was a Friday. My day would be on the weekend for the first time in a long time. I didn't want to give him Sunday after the big day had already passed. My son-shine was all dressed up too. Black pants and a long-sleeved black button-up. We rode an hour to Baltimore to a new fine-dining vegan restaurant. They gave us a white quartz stone with our receipt. Issa said he felt like royalty, like a king, because of it. This experience raised his dining expectations.

Saturday morning, I had day-long plans with the girls. This year, we did a spa in DC, a brunch at a hotel, and Swingers the Crazy Golf Club, an indoor putting spot for adults. I sure wish I vetted that spa in advance. It was small, and one of the massage rooms had workout equipment in the massage room. When one person was paying for their service, the entire cash register kiosk fell apart. My four-twenty-friendly friend appreciated that this spa was focused on the healing power of CBD and sold several infused CBD items, including drinks, oils, and soaps. Brunch was coincidentally where my friend who came from out of town was staying, which was convenient. Swingers was where all the fun went down. The package that we purchased came with four drink tickets each.

SWG made a surprise appearance and played golf with us. I asked him to play golf in my honor, as my arm was still hurting from surgery. Naturally, all the girls asked who he was, and I said that's my friend. Followed by, "Ooooo." I was like, "No, like a plutonic friend, not friend-friend." He mentioned something about still communicating with his ex, and I don't think he was into me. They teased, like Girl, whatever. He is looking at you in that dress. My brunch dress was black with lace mesh in the middle; it was fire.

CHAPTER 4

SEPTEMBER 2020
SUPERWOMAN
(THREE YEARS)

The day started with a ring at the doorbell. Flowers from my sister. Issa and I spent most of the day at home. I didn't have too much in me this year. I really wanted to be in bed; I didn't push myself hard. Quantico Park had made some upgrades, and I made sure to visit in time to catch the sunset. There was a lovely patio and a café. Issa and I watched the water and chatted at the café table.

I started Self-Care September for myself in 2019 for multiple reasons. It was the anniversary of my mom's passing, and I noticed how much I hadn't cared for myself in the past few years. To the point of actually losing a tooth! Self-care can be comprehensive and time-consuming. Upon research, I discovered September is indeed Self-Care Awareness Month, founded in 2017.

I started my self-care process in August this year in honor of the month I was born and my own existence. Although self-care August doesn't rhyme at all, it seemed appropriate to do a few cosmetic things in time for August 28, such as laser hair removal. My skin was glowing, and I was smooth as a baby everywhere, but I knew I needed to dig deeper and continue to make appointments to check out my health, as well as attend therapy regularly through September. This year, it was a sixty-day process.

On September 12, I had a terrible accident. I planned to trim the trees while Issa learned to ride his bike. I turned on IG Live to show how to trim my bushes, something I have done a million times before. Within a minute, I started the hedge cutter with my hand in the wrong place and cut through my finger. I quietly turned off the Live and screamed. I was in so much pain. I ran to get a bag of ice.

I told Issa, "Drop the bike and let's go." I drove to the ER feeling that I would pass out or throw up. I was in a rush and the ER was not. They gave me a throw-up bag that I didn't need while I rotted in the waiting room.

They called me to the back, where I waited a million hours and years. I went between crying and staring into space. Eventually, they gave me an injection that made my finger feel like a big balloon and put stitches in. I could not fucking believe it. I was mad at everything, mad I went outside, mad I was on Live, mad I tried to do three things at once, mad I cut my finger.

When I got home, Issa's orange Mongoose bike was thrown down in front of the house. The blood in the sink from when I tried to rinse my finger looked like something disastrous happened. I was morose. I went to my bed. I posted about it the next day. I also finished cutting the bushes just to show myself I could. No one visited, and I didn't feel better after completing the job.

I found the following words in my notepad that I used as a diary at the time. Dated September 16, 2021. It was a short poem, "Superwoman," and a long entry titled, My Feelings in English:

My feelings in a poem.

"Superwoman"

Superwoman is dead

She tried to carry the world, but instead,

she dropped it on her head

But no one on Earth noticed she was down

Because the world crushed her skull without making a sound

She screamed for help, and no one could hear her

She was in space, light years away with no supplies

Her life was flashing before her eyes

An indication she would die

The bird that rose from ashes born of the sun

Was all depleted and finally done

Her heart was named Issa

The gift from Saturn

Got lost in a confusing pattern

The journey between love, hate, abandonment, and hope

Made no sense, like a goat in a coat

With no map to navigate the way

The heart had no direction and could not stay

Issa and Superwoman went away

My Feelings in English

Coming home and seeing everything as I left it made me feel sad. I didn't feel strong and independent. I feel burned out, undesirable, and unprotected.

SWG went on a trip for two weeks. I have not done any martial arts in a while, which was my usual release. I saw how well-dressed he was on this trip, and it reassured me of what I already knew about men in love. He came to my birthday in some Nike shoes; he showed up to that birthday in Prada shoes. But deeper than material things—where is the person who wants to dress up for me and take a plane to come to where I am? Does love have a limit? After you pass up the first few people that try, do you get no more?

October 10 will make three years of no sex by choice because I feel like anyone will fuck me, but no one I'm attracted to loves me. I've had my share of guys taking me on dates, but I don't want to exploit anyone for food. I just want to love someone and be loved back. It sounds so simple and seems impossible.

I thought that I accepted the fact that perhaps there was no match for me, but it really sucks when something bad happens and there is no one to lean on. No one to watch my son on my birthday or ride bikes with him.

My mom was rigid with me, but she was supportive, and now I am a shoe with no sole. I feel every piece of dirt and chewed gum as I try to navigate life, and I'm so tired—eighty-three-year-old-woman tired. I'm thirty-eight but feel eighty-three.

Believing things would get better always kept me going; believing I could figure anything out always gave me hope. But the one thought: *What if things stay just like this; what if I never figure it out? Then what?*

I had a bunch of degrees from a bunch of average ass institutions and I felt mediocre. Very not enough. Very Whitney Houston. Didn't we almost have it all? While I am on track to finding another decent job, how long before they fire me like all the others?

Where the fuck do I belong? I do not have the resources to roll out some of my visions, and my energy keeps going missing.

I have done so many things, and while some were impactful and memorable, the mix of longevity and lack of monetary stability makes everything feel like a failure. It was done, but what does it lead to?? Where is the big bang?? The mountain top??

My dad says you cannot win a race if you give up, so I stay in the race, but can you win the race if you are slow? Can you win the race if you think you won, then got tested and failed and got stripped like Sha'Carri Richardson?

One day, I felt like the baddest, most unfuckable-with woman. The next, I felt unseen and short of whatever is required to be a provider and a sturdy foundation for at least my son. Everything is too heavy. I've been hating mom'ing. I suppose there was a loss of control and comfort. My kid was home, and then he was released to school. Where kids threw his eraser away, called him coronavirus, and teased him about his hair. I will fuck all those kids up. Issa came home with his hair down because the kids talked about his hairstyle. First of all, the bun keeps his hair out of his face, and second, my finger is cut, and I can't change the style, and that made me feel kind of bad.

For the past forty-eight hours, I have been struggling. I've been so annoyed by my son. He doesn't listen, ever, and the thoughts of not wanting to be a mom anymore make me feel guilty and terrible. I don't feel the joy. It is just annoying, every second of it. Repeating myself, cooking in pain, cleaning in pain.

It seems like I made one mistake—picking an irresponsible father—and I am going to be punished with no support as though he is actually dead for the rest of my life. Issa's kid years are half over. No stepdad ever stepped in. He has never seen me be loved. I hate it.

I felt like we were so special, just the two of us, and on closer review, it feels like we are both not shit and not going to be shit. If I don't give 110 percent, my son won't be able to maintain his academics, and I don't have the energy. Basically, once I chill, Issa will become a bum. I just can't. I am tired, and it doesn't seem like a weekend or yoga classes will fix it.

I need a fucking actual other parent, our person. I need fucking help, and help is not coming, so I feel overwhelmed. I'm very disappointed my mind isn't strong enough to believe that I can do anything. I somehow have been catapulted into a crippling and hopeless frame of thought.

I don't like speaking about it to those around me. I get this feeling that even with the few I speak to, they don't have the capacity to care that much because they have their own life shit and their own families to deal with.

My brother's hardship didn't help. I can hear that coming home was always his first solution to problems. Just the fear of living together puts me in a slight panic attack, but maybe I am overthinking it.

I miss Classic Man, and I wish someone had feelings for me the way I have feelings for him. A loveless life is more painful than my fucking finger right now. Luckily, Tylenol helps with heartbreak, although it can only be treated for six hours at a time.

༺✿༻

I was going through it. I was spiraling the drain quickly. I watched *The White Lotus* for comedic relief and *The Sweet Life*. Then I binge-watched *Mare of Eastown,* especially at night. On the eighteenth, my cousin had a baby shower; I couldn't go out looking like my feelings. I threw on some makeup and a smile and went back outside. September 23, Dad sent me pictures of Grandma. She had a lovely pink and white cake and a pink ribbon that said Party Girl.

September 25. Issa and I were invited for an overnight stay at MGM because Erykah was in town for her Badubatron tour stop. It had been two years since Issa had attended a live concert. He was ecstatic. He enjoyed the lighting sequences during the performance, watching Frank Moka play the drums up close, and felt like a very special person. The highlight of his night: the logo maracas that Erykah gifted him. They lit up and made noise. I was sure that I would get a seizure from how much he was shaking them.

After the concert, the late night was mine. Issa watched TV and played games in the room, and my cousin and I hit the casino and nightlife. I had so much fun that night. Dancing and two-stepping, eating, and laughing. It was a huge relief from my everyday life. I was so grateful that we were all together and that I was invited. Sometimes, bringing your kid is a deal breaker, and I was happy that I made bringing him a regular thing. It was expected for him to be there.

I did my first Hair Therapy Pop-Up in October in front of My Mama's Vegan. I had the idea to let Issa sell his cookies, "Prince Issa's Vegan Cookies" with me. His cookies sold out in fifteen to twenty minutes, and he made $42 while I sat there with bottles of oil, lol. I sold more than I would have online, about eight bottles. It was a good first experience, but Issa didn't feel so hot. His eye was swollen. The struggles of a child with telegenic and bountiful eyelashes, and he wanted to go home as soon as he got there. He was not impressed by his success.

Another encouraging and funny thing happened—I received a birthday gift in October. It was a bag with a coconut hibiscus candle, a wooden box with a clock on the outside, bath soap, shampoo, conditioner and lotion, a silver ring, and a book, *Breaking Night* by Liz Murray. A personable card and chocolate. My spirits were lifted.

The gift gave me enough energy to continue with my job search. I applied to Howard University for Communication Associate and other positions and Amazon for Product Marketing Manager and Marketing Manager to Underserved Populations. I was hopeful.

In the meantime, I selected my participants for RAE2022, and it was time to record interviews and do photoshoots. This was my favorite part of the process because the men usually get to meet each other. This time was different; the schedules would not come together, and we had to do each one individually. One interview was scheduled for December and two for January, which was crazy because all three participants were usually shot in October so that I had all the months I needed to edit.

The most monumental thing that happened was that my dad sent me a picture on October 27, 2021, and it was a gold bracelet with my name on it. On his trip to Guyana, he had a new one made for me, and I was pleased. It is noticeably different than the first one; the letters were smaller, and the design was completely different. I felt complete again. It meant so much to me that Dad went the extra mile to have it replaced. My heart was full.

In November, I was placed on 15 mg of Mirtazapine. Mirtazapine is an antidepressant used to treat major depressive disorder in adults. Some of the side effects are worse than what it cures. For me, it caused stomach cramps. I was crippled under financial pressure. I quit styling in July; it was November! I hadn't been offered a position yet. My therapist recommended getting a loan for my business. The process was lengthy, but I did not let it discourage me. I applied on November 18, 2021 and was approved for $15,000.

I needed to understand what was going on with my son, so I took him for psychological testing. After a series of tests, it was determined that he had ADHD. This affected his executive functioning skills and led to disorder and disorganization, which was one of the reasons his desk at school and room at home were so messy. The Dr. told me it could get worse as he gets older. He recommended that Issa be given extra time to finish assignments and an agenda.

I couldn't make it to see Dad for his birthday (November 5) this year. Aunty Roxy had a lovely black and gold birthday party on November 10. Issa played "My Heart Will Go On" by Celine Dionne for her and she cried. It was sublime. Aunty also hosted Thanksgiving. Many of my cousins were there, including Zaria. This was where the first discussion of making a coloring book for the cognitive distortions mentioned in *Beautiful Reject* started. I also drew a lot this month, sketching ideas for a product line and what the packaging would look like.

Winter

In December, I had a surprise birthday party for my sister, and everyone came—our cousins, usually in Cali, my friend who lived in New York, and my Hair Therapy birthday group. This was the year I made my infamous seventeen-pound crispy-skin turkey. Everyone was raving about how juicy and amazing it was. Two things made that turkey special. First, it was given to me by my therapist. She always had my family in mind with resources beyond talk therapy. Second, I am vegan and did not taste it. I cooked it from memory using a recipe from 2010.

December was SWG's birthday, and I planned a trip to the range and lunch. It was my thank you for all the Saturdays of working out together. Our theme seemed to be all about safety, and guns were something that I had more experience with. Issa played Happy Birthday for him when we returned, and it seemed he had a good time.

During the holidays, I like to keep it really chill to work on upcoming projects in peace. Shooting participant one in December went well. Issa was on the set, and I felt how important it was for him to be present during these moments. I made a conscious decision that I would bring him to the recordings of all the interviews.

The top of January shooting of participant two went well, and then I was hit with the news that participant three could not come to Woodbridge. He was working on a TV show. It was great that he was doing amazing things, but I panicked because my photographer wasn't available to go to New York with me to shoot him. I was stressed. This man was already on a hit show on ABC, and I am going to New York to shoot him on my A6000! OMG. Death by imposter syndrome. I booked a studio and did my best, but every fiber of my being wished that Kevin or my sister— you know, the fucking professionals—were there! Issa was there, and that really lightened my nerves. They took selfies, and I was just amazed at how he connected with everyone.

When it was time to edit and integrate my Sony footage with Kevin's Black magic footage and beast-ass audio footage,

I wanted to scream into my pillow. Capturing him was better than not getting the interview at all, but it didn't compare to my producer's work. I wanted perfection.

The most emotional part of this RAE was that one of the intended participants died before he could do his interview. Chef Rob was the chef for the RAE2020 dinner; he told me, "This is dope; I want to be on the big screen next time." I texted him in October and was supposed to give him a call the next day. I did not call him, and he passed away later that week. It took the wind out of me. I opened the documentary with a tribute to him and wished I had reached out sooner so his family could hear him tell his story. I also felt horrible for not calling in general when I said I would. Chef Rob was my inspiration to leave creative, intimate venues and present my film in the movie theater for the first time. He said the big screen, and I took it literally.

RAE2022

During the month of February, we were hustling for our lives. Issa was selling cookies online, playing the guitar every day on Live, and reading Black History facts. I applied for a one-time bailout plan at Social Services. The program pays two bills that you are behind on. I was waiting impatiently for my taxes. I applied for so many jobs that I had a spreadsheet. I finally had a somewhat reasonable offer, but with all good jobs, the onboarding process takes forever, and you may be dead by the time they call you to coordinate a start date. They called me while I was at the Alamo doing a sound check for RAE. They told me things were all set, and I started the following week. I was able to go into the event with less stress. I was baffled at how I went through the same shit every time I put on this show. No money, no job, filing taxes—did I not pass the test of fortitude the first time?

SWG attended the event dressed in a black suit with a tie and made a nice donation. I took note of that. I sat next to him when I could. I had two guests who were not dressed up, and I thought to myself, *For my next show, I'm getting bouncers.* Issa made a brief appearance on screen when he received his gift of chopsticks from Malik DOPE. The crowd aww'd, and his eyeballs popping out from seeing himself onscreen was such a mom moment for me.

This event took a lot to put together, which is why I have it every other year. In 2022, I scheduled it on the repunit date of February 2, 2022, and I preplanned the next one for February 24, 2024, and the one after that on February 26, 2026. I will run out of cool dates in 2028 (February 28, 2028). Why do the dates matter? For me, it boils down to memory and archiving. I can't tell you when the first (2018) and second (2020) RAEs were held without looking them up because those dates had no pizzazz.

It was March 1, my first day at the new job, and I got a text asking if I wanted to return to my old job. The irony. I had to call to confirm, "Are you serious?" Yes, we are putting a team together; we have room and money for you. I took a $20,000 pay cut for the new job I was in. It was a no-brainer that I wanted to go back. To not be hasty, I waited until my old job called with an official new start date.

I continued working and was looking forward to the opportunity to go back to my old team. I was ripped from them suddenly, and it sucked. I can count on one hand how many times I gave a shit about a job—twice—my job at the University with my mentor and this one. It's not really the job but the connection and the respect for the person that extended the opportunity. The university gave me knowledge of how educational institutions and boards work. The financial impact was not life-changing, but knowledge and working with my mentor before he retired was invaluable.

This opportunity taught me about IT, and the money was life-changing. It allowed me to be current with a cushion and think about options I didn't have in the past. The timeline of survival mode, from employed to unemployed, to entrepreneur to loan, and to being employed with a pay cut, taught me a lot. I vowed that if I could get back in, I would do it all. I would pay things off, travel, save, get a house, and I would not let anyone tell me what I could or could not do. I would give it my best effort.

I had a notepad that I started during COVID-19 with a list of places I wanted to visit, and everything shut down before I could go anywhere. I erased the year 2020 and renamed the list "reworked from 2020." I added RAE2022 and placed a little check on it. I needed a sense of accomplishment. I added dates in the future to destinations already listed and told myself these plans were delayed but right on time. They will happen. I started extensively researching hotels and points of interest all over the world. I would spend hours creating itineraries for places I had no tickets for.

Later in March, I took a day trip to Philly to explore the vegan food options and view the Harriet Tubman "The Journey to Freedom" sculpture that was there for a limited time. This was the day I realized how much I craved to be connected to Black History or water in all my travels. We finished the month by visiting the Tubman Museum in Roanoke, Virginia. I drove four hours from my house to show Issa the original Black Panther costume. Other awesome displays included the clothing from *Coming to America*, Spike Lee's *Do the Right Thing*, and *Malcolm X*.

This trip was challenging because my hand was swollen, and my stomach was hurting. I was fine the day before and the day after. Sometimes I get that sense that a force is trying to deter me, and when I feel that feeling, I push harder. Issa and I think so differently; he was most impressed with King James' (LeBron James) outfit for Fortnite's Icon Series on display created by Ruth E. Carter. Lebron James is his favorite basketball player.

April is for Issa 2022

For Issa's tenth birthday, I decorated downstairs with a Miles Morales Spider-Man theme. I had been collecting his custom gifts for weeks: a Miles Morales phone case, Miles Morales shirts, a bracelet made for him, and red cupcakes. I do well with wrapped gifts, but for the big ten, I wanted more decorations. There was an easel with a costume sign that read Happy Tenth with the Spider-Man font with his picture below making the Spider-Man gesture. Black and red balloons everywhere.

A week or so prior, his dad called asking if I had plans for him, and I said, "Of course. You have never had a birthday with him ever; why are you trying to start now? This is also the tenth parenting anniversary, and I don't want to share it with you."

My aunt told me that I was harsh, and she thought that Issa would really enjoy seeing his dad. I tried to wrap my head around it. Can I do this? Generally, most people would say a child needs their dad. I have a great relationship and cannot imagine a life without my dad. What I am not sure is needed is a person that pops up out of nowhere and disappears. It causes the child to be extremely happy and then extremely sad. That low is hard to watch. I had already been through it time and time again with Issa. I knew he would be pumped for the high, but could he handle the low? It was such a tough decision.

One of the inside jokes is that Issa thinks his dad looks like Spider-Man because he is so fit. When he received the action figure some time ago, I asked him who it looked like to him. He said, Dad. He wasn't wrong, but in a way, that was dangerous. We want our parents to be our heroes, but can we maintain that image when they do not show up? Heroes show up.

With that trailing thought, I said, "You can be Spider-Man; he would probably like that if he is not terrified." He said OK. He said he ordered the costume and sent a picture. All I could do was blink. That is Peter Parker. I said, "Why the fuck are you Peter Parker, navy and red? I said Miles Morales, Spider-Man, is black and red. I was so annoyed that I didn't even want him to come anymore.

During Issa's family birthday FaceTime, there was some excitement about Spider-Man being on the call. Issa seemed so shy and a little confused; his face screamed, *How did my mom get Spider-Man to come to my house?* When the call was over, I said, "Issa, who is that?" He said, "I don't know." His dad took his mask off and he said, "DAD!" and gave him a hug.

It was a tender moment, but it still pissed me off inside. I could see that Issa wasn't ready because he wasn't expecting this reunion, and it was a lot to take in. They ate cupcakes. I let them chat, and we took him to school. That was the only time he had been taken to school by both of his parents. The day was marvelous and such a facade. A reality only made possible by this special day. From this day, Issa finally has a picture with him and both of his parents. Something that should not be so hard to come by.

In the afternoon, we greeted him when he came home from school. His dad helped him get dressed for his formal dinner. We said goodbye and headed to Aunty Roxy's and then to Double Zero in Baltimore. Double Zero was a vegan upscale restaurant that offered pizza. They put a ten on his pizza, and I've never seen a smile so big. The day, the effort, patience, and tolerance were worth it.

I got the call that April 18 was my new start at my old job. I was already on a pre-approved vacation time for April 11-15 and was bursting with nerves about delivering the resignation. They did the shadiest thing—they asked me to adjust my notice to April 8 and then tried to withhold my PTO. That was laughable. I complained that it was underhanded of HR, and they paid it out.

For Issa's tenth birthday, I also planned a big surprise. I booked a trip to Iceland and Minnesota in the same week. After Issa had his guitar lesson on Monday, April 11, we headed to the airport. He loved airplanes and was curious about where we were headed. When I got to the Iceland Air counter, there was no one there, and we missed check-in time. I made a bunch of calls to no avail. He cried at the airport. I cried at the airport, and we went home. I told him we would be heading to Minnesota in a few days because Mommy planned two trips, which helped with the tears. I booked a nonrefundable flight to Iceland, rationalizing that there was no way I would ever miss my flight. When I was unable to get a refund for the Iceland trip, it hurt so much. The same with the hotels. I felt like an idiot.

The trip to Minnesota was a do-over because, on our road trip around the US, I messed up big time. I didn't purchase the tickets to Paisley Park in advance, and we could not get in. We were only able to go to the gift shop, which was a huge disappointment. For this do-over trip, I bought the VIP tickets before I even booked the flight. I booked a nice hotel and a rental and made sure I had all the details covered. Dad flew in from New York, and we flew in from DC. The tour was great.

My dad enjoyed it. We saw Prince's extensive shoe collection and stood in studios where he made classics. We saw the Purple Rain bike. It was really cool. This was one time that I was happy; I was a person that overdoes it. Issa still whispered about Iceland in the upcoming weeks, and I told him to zip it—enough—we are moving on.

When I returned to work, things were different. Training was set up to be vigorous and more efficient. I was working, working. It made me wonder what exactly I was doing before. After about a month, we had an in-person lunch, and it was nice to see everyone. I still got invited to the lunches when I didn't work there, but it felt good to be officially on the team and not on the outside looking in.

I had papers scattered all across my room, figuring out how to adult better. I did not want to overwhelm myself. I started with the basics, putting everything on auto-pay. That was a big step. My new pay structure was once a month, so there was no point in playing around. If I did not pay something, it would be a month late. When I shared with someone that I was paid monthly, he said, "That once a month will either mess you up or make you really responsible," and I wanted to be on the really responsible side.

I received a text from Ms. Bentley saying that I needed to get Issa. She heard that something was happening at the school. When I arrived, the police were outside and not letting anyone out of the building. I was scared. I spoke to SWG as I waited for details. I was trembling. Eventually, the assistant principal told me that Issa was not at school. He evacuated the building and would be brought back shortly by a bus. I was very concerned; evacuated to where and why?

When the bus arrived, the kids came off the bus crying, and the teacher was crying. Issa ran to me and started telling me what happened. Someone broke into the school, broke into his classroom, the principal came in to try to stop her, and she assaulted the principal. During the attack, Issa and his class ran out of the back door to the nearest recreation center and sheltered in place until they received word that it was safe to return. Of all the schools and all the classrooms, why was this crazy lady at my son's school? He spoke about it for weeks, and the experience shattered the notion that school was a safe place for him.

Juneteenth was on the horizon. I did not learn about Juneteenth until I was an adult, and this was the first time it would be recognized as a federal holiday. I would be in New York for my cousin's birthday and Father's Day. I signed up for a basketball workshop for Issa. A player from the WNBA Liberty team showed him the basics. He was gifted a Brooklyn Nets basketball, but the best part of the day was meeting John Starks. As a kid, I had his basketball card, and I thought he was so cute back when he played with Patrick Ewing. I never owned a pair of the 33 Hi's or the Reebok Pumps, but they were cool too. My dad watched all the home games. He has the Knicks glasses, mugs, cups, and pencils. Seeing Mr. Starks took me back to that time in life.

I wanted to show Dad some appreciation because it had been a long road. When Dad's phone rang and my name came across his screen, he never knew what he would hear on the other end. I took him and my brother to the Polo Bar in Manhattan. We were noticeably the only Black patrons there. My brother ordered fruit punch, and I wanted to spit out my water. I thought to myself, *Does this look like the type of place where you can order some damn fruit punch?*

Watching the sever say, "We don't have fruit punch" was like watching a person speak in slow motion. Dad's cheesecake said Happy Father's Day! And his gift was a Polo travel bag. What inspired this experience was a bottle of cologne. Growing up, my dad always had a bottle of Polo cologne in the green glass bottle with a gold top. Somewhere in the past ten years, it changed to the red bottle. The brand loyalty was real. Hence, the Polo-themed day. When he read his card and saw the step repeat logo, he said, "Wait a minute. I think you have a theme here," and I smiled.

Ms. Bentley recommended Issa to a young scholar's program. They offered him a partial scholarship to attend a weeklong camp at the University of Carolina Chapel Hill. Even with the scholarship, the camp cost over $1,000. I was on the fence about it, but I wanted him to have new experiences. We shared the news with social media and the Hair Therapy tribe. He received $400 the day the word got out. I paid for the rest in a few monthly installments. I read about the program, and some said it was an over-glorified summer camp. Personally, I wanted to make sure I followed every lead sent his way by the educator who believed in him. I want them to know we value their referrals and guidance.

On the first day of camp, we arrived early and went to our favorite café, COCO, where we discovered our waterfall adventures. I spent the first night at a nearby hotel. He called and said he didn't have lotion, and I dropped some off. I was speaking to a friend, and she said, "Some parents are in Paris. Go home."

I wasn't ready to leave, so I went to the spa. It was called Skin Sense. It had a salt room with lots of pink salt on the floor. I wasn't sure how this was supposed to be healing, but I was there to try new things and took a seat. The session was thirty minutes. I sat down, and a minute later, a staff member tapped me on the shoulder, telling me that thirty minutes was up. What?

How did I fall asleep so fast? It was the deepest, best sleep. I have been to other salt rooms that have salt on the walls with no loose salt on the floor, and it just is not the same.

Next, I had a massage that felt so good. The song from *Scandal* was playing, "The Light," and The Album Leaf's "Into the Blue Again." I did not expect that. I was in tears. Some people hated that show, but I know that Oliva and Fitz feeling, and ugh, I wouldn't wish it on my worst enemies. I only heard the song when watching the show; I never heard it on the radio. I wasn't ready to get hit with the Olitz soundtrack.

August—a family trip to Jamaica was in the works for a year. I could not do the payment plan that everyone else was doing when the emails initially rolled out. Now that the departure date was approaching, I didn't want to miss the opportunity to bask in the sun with my Aunty Roxy. I was recently approved for a credit card and ready to put it to good use. I grabbed two tickets for Issa and me and booked a three-day stay. I paid more than everyone else because my purchase was last minute, and I was OK with that. I made sure that I was ready early and on time at the airport.

We were off to Jamaica. Issa said, "Mom, we did it; we finally left America." I laughed. The funniest part of the trip was his commentary on the planes. "Mom, this is an older model. Mom, that was a hard landing." Issa really thought he was the Rotten Tomatoes of aircraft experiences.

Once we arrived, I declared that the day was his and the night was mine. We spent the day in the sun and hanging out by the pool. At night, I went to the resort clubs. I learned there was a vegan place in Negril on Seven-Mile Beach. I hired a driver to take us. The beach was full of hustlers trying to sell us stuff every second. We were not dropped off at the closest entrance, and it felt like we walked miles to get to this place. By the time I saw the sign, I thought it was a mirage. I ordered everything and ate everything. The wildest part of this adventure was finding out that the slushies I gave Issa had liquor at the end of the trip.

Going home, I used a long layover in Orlando to visit Disney Springs and spend the night in a hotel connected to the airport. A guy approached me after leaving the immigration line. I thought I heard him say something in the line.

He said, "I said you're beautiful."

I said, "Thank you," and he asked for my number. That night, he kept asking when he could see me. I said I have my son; I can't see you. Then he offered to visit me at the hotel. He was trying to hook up even though I was with my son. I didn't like that. Once we returned home, we spoke on a few FaceTimes here and there, and as the details unfolded, things got worse. He said he was doing Amazon deliveries for work, and after a week, he told me I wasn't acting like I wanted to be in a relationship. The final straw was when he asked me to look for flights so he could come and surprise Issa. This man was delusional on the next level, and I know these lines actually worked on someone in the past.

I tuned him out and worked on upgrading my room. I removed the popcorn ceiling, changed the beige walls to white, and added a black access wall on the left. I got the black wall idea from a picture I found in my mom's magazines that she starred and labeled bedroom. This was one of my gifts to myself—creating a sanctuary. I rebuilt the bookshelves and painted them black back in June. The look was coming together. The space was starting to look designed.

August is for Me 2023

My birthday slogan this year was Aiming to Relax. Starting the morning at the range and ending it at the spa. Our group had a private room with three lanes. There was a mix of first-timers and regulars. We were shooting at 9 a.m. Gangbanging over breakfast. When we were done, we went to Lansdowne Resort. I went to see in advance if it was large enough to accommodate all of us. I arrived and she said the spa pool was broken. I wanted to knock her register over. Why is there some type of issue at these spas on my day? The ladies reported that they liked the relaxation rooms and the services they selected. For the jacuzzi, we had to go up a whole floor and pass a gym. It was not the elite experience I planned, but the ladies made jokes about everything, and we had fun. I was smiling and happy to be around my people. We don't see each other often, but we carve out the time once a year to get together. The day serves two purposes: one is celebrating making it another year, and the other is sisterhood and motherhood.

CHAPTER 5

SEPTEMBER 2022 - JANUARY 2023

HAPPY TO STUPID

(FOUR YEARS, FOUR MONTHS)

Four long years since Mom had been away, and this year, I didn't want to run. No road trip, no waterfalls. Home improvement was top of mind.

I had a vision to create a family art wall and needed a chic, clean hallway. This was "the hallway project"—removing popcorn from the hallways and the steps. It took me days; I started on the first and didn't finish until the third. Phase one was scraping, sanding, painting, then painting again. I looked through Issa's and my sister's art, picked my favorites, and hung them up. I had a few contributions also. The cherry on top was that I found the perfect place to put my mom's picture—right over the staircase so you could see it when you went down the stairs.

Moving mom's pictures was significant. I had two big photos of her in my room from her memorial. One was on the left side of the bed and the other on the right. The way my bed is set up, the pillows against the headboard are in front of the black curtains where the window is. If I sleep the way the bed is made, I often catch a cold or wake up with a sore throat. One day, I decided to sleep the opposite way with my head away from the window, and I woke up not feeling like I was on the brink of a cold. That became my regular evening routine. When

I sleep upside down and open my eyes, Mom's picture is the first thing I see. Like in *50 First Dates,* seeing those pictures is how my brain remembered she was gone. It's how I came out of shock and disbelief.

When I was shooting a promo video for my book, I swapped Mom's photos with identical framed covers of my coloring book. I put one of her photos in the guest room. Mainly family visits me, and they are always happy to see the big picture of her there. I placed the other in the hallway. I liked that the repositioning allowed everyone to see her, and I also was taking steps to be comfortable in a room that was once hers.

Shortly after the project was complete, I rallied the Hair Therapy ladies together for a day of empowerment. The long-awaited movie *The Woman King* was in theaters. It was based on a true story. In the 1800s, a group of all-female warriors protected the African kingdom of Dahomey with skills and fierceness unlike anything the world has ever seen. Faced with a new threat, General Nanisca trains the next generation of recruits to fight against a foreign enemy that's determined to destroy their way of life.

I enjoyed watching this film because I felt seen and understood. It showed a woman's ability to fight, plan, sacrifice, and rejoice. While I am not a warrior, I identify with the concept of going against the grain and the burden of being responsible for multiple people's livelihoods. The film reminds us that all women don't solve problems in a mild-mannered fashion, and sometimes, compliance is not enough to get the job done. Watching *The Woman King* with a group of amazing African American women really made it one of the most memorable movie experiences.

Grandma's Birthday 2022

It was September 23, 2022 and time to visit the woman king of my family, Grandma. She turned the big ninety this year. When I saw the outfit, she was going to wear, I declared to my dad it was not fancy enough. It needed to be fabulous. She was going to be 90. Grandma lost her sight, and I had to describe her dress. She could tell it was fancy and wanted makeup. That made me smile, and I put some powder on her cheeks. My dad went to the store and came back with a striking black and gold horizontally striped dress. The dress matched Issa's black and gold bow tie, and I wore a black velvet dress.

I captured an image of Issa standing and smiling with Grandma smiling behind him. Grandma had her crown on, and I need to applaud Dad for getting the little birthday accessories she has every year. They are so cute. I was happy for her, and I wrote this tribute for her in the September Newsletter.

My grandma, Marian Hopkinson, was born in Guyana, South America, on September 23, 1932. She married my grandfather, Lionel Hopkinson, and moved to America in 1977 when she was forty-five. She was a midwife in Guyana, and to continue that work in the US, she worked as a home health aide and acquired a GED.

Eventually, she became a pediatric nurse at North Shore Hospital in Manhasset, New York. Grandma worked the overnight shift. She left at 9 p.m. every night and took several buses with a travel time of over an hour.

In 1987, she purchased a new construction home in Brooklyn, New York. I was four years old, and I remember the fence being installed and the trees being planted.

In 2007, she retired from North Shore Hospital after thirty years of service and has since traveled to Africa and her home country. In 2010, she transferred ownership of her home to her son, Dale Hopkinson (my dad) and granddaughter (me).

Currently, in 2022, Marian is ninety years old. She still lives at 1936 and enjoys listening to her great-grandson, Issa Hopkinson, play the guitar when he visits.

I accompanied her bio with photos from her younger days and nursing days. While writing her bio, I realized I wanted to be like my grandma. I wanted to buy a house, and I wanted it to be new. I want a place that can provide solace for my child and his children. I had been an entrepreneur for years and wasn't pulling in enough to get approved for a house in my area. To reach the requirements in a timely fashion, I focused on obtaining two years of W-2s. By April 2024, I would be eligible. That was the motivation. If Grandma can work for thirty years, I can work for two. Going forward, I took better digital and written notes to improve at work to learn and understand the job. I changed my mindset from this is just a job to I need this job to get this house. I paid more attention, gave useful feedback, and asked more questions.

To be resourceful and responsible, I continued to thrift. It was one of my mom's favorite pastimes. Sometimes, I would shop by myself and look up and see her. The best surprise ever. She would always find me something. She had the best eye. After losing her, I didn't go to the thrift store for a while. It was not as fun without her, and knowing I would never bump into her while shopping again was crushing. On this day, I went in good spirits, thinking mom would want me to save money and buy things I needed. I found a Badgley Mischka purse with a broken buckle, and I couldn't put it down. I had the idea to take it to Bedo, the leather man, to see if it could be restored. That worked out well, and he told me the purse was a good find.

October was about restoring and preserving, and my next mini project was the kitchen ceiling. It took two days to remove the popcorn from the ceiling and paint it white. It is a mystery why the ceiling in the kitchen is so low. This worked to my advantage when I was standing, saving me from stretching and hurting my arms.

I had two very memorable moments in October; the first was celebrating a Hair Therapy member's fiftieth birthday. It was nice to be invited to something so important and intimate. It was a dinner with her closest friends, one of whom I connected with immediately. She was so easygoing, and it felt like I had known her forever, although I had never seen her in my life. I was disappointed when she said she lived in North Carolina.

The second most memorable moment was going to Iceland. I managed to book and coordinate a second trip for Issa and me. This time, I was incredibly early to the airport. I went to Ms. Vicky at Sunshine Nails for some long white nails. A sure sign that I planned to do no hard work on the trip. Being pretty and taking in the sights would be my full-time job. I had been researching for months and found all the good vegan places to eat. I made plans to visit the south. It takes seven days to circle Ring Road, and we only had three to spare.

As soon as we stepped off the plane, we rented a car and headed to the Blue Lagoon. My first panic attack was being separated from my son. He could not come into the locker room with me. I had to send him and his luggage to the men's locker room, and staff escorted him. We met in the main area and entered the lagoon. It was foggy, mystical, and the most stirring thing I have ever seen. The mountains were in the distance. The sun was out, the water, which looked like blue milk, was warm, and the air was cold. So many things happened at once; I recorded holding my son's hand.

In that moment, I was full of joy. I thought to myself, *Pinch me this can't be real.* I see why so many people have flocked here, and I can't get down my IG timeline without seeing a girls' group post that they were in Iceland. I longed for no one. I was with my favorite person. I made my favorite person, raised him, and then brought him on vacation! I am amazing. We are amazing, and no one else matters. We stayed for hours. We did the mud masks, and I had my first water massage.

When we went to dine at lunch, a lady kept looking at me and smiling. I wasn't sure what she was smiling for. I assumed she was smiling because she was looking at the two happiest glowing people in the room. When we finished dessert, the server said our bill had been paid. That has never happened before. A bill covered by a stranger. It was a kind gesture that made my heart warm. They didn't say one word to us directly. Her generosity started my visit on a high note.

After visiting the Blue Lagoon, we reset at our first hotel. I rewashed each of our heads with products for afro hair to prevent damage. First thing in the morning, we followed Ring Road southeast toward Vik. After spending a few hours in Vik for lunch, it was tempting to hang out until check-in; however, I continued driving further southeast to the Jökulsárlón Glacier Lagoon. We caught the best view just before sunset.

Following the Jökulsárlón excursion, we returned to Vik for much-needed rest at hotel number two. We had no luck seeing the Northern Lights on the two-and-a-half-hour drive back from the glacier lagoon or overnight! Instead, we were greeted with hail and Icelandic wind. The wind was so aggressive that it moved our bodies as we walked. I hoped and wished the Northern lights would make an appearance, but they never did. I selected the modern Kria Hotel because of its ceiling-to-floor walls in the hope that we would be looking at the Northern Lights all night. Instead, we made dance videos, and I taught Issa to play pool in the recreation room. It felt like we were up all night giggling and roaming around; we had no interest in sleeping.

On day three, we visited Black Sand Beach before leaving Vik. It flipped my brain inside out, seeing the black sand as far as the eye could see. The *Game of Thrones* intro played endlessly in my head. It looked like I rented the beach just for us. I didn't see many people there. Then we followed Ring Road back toward the capital. We stopped to see two waterfalls coming from the south heading north. The first was **Skógafoss**; you can walk right up to it. It was grand. Tons of white water crashing into dark black sand. The sound of the water is everything a meditation tape tries to capture. There was zero railing if you wanted to jump in and end it all; you were free to go. If you got too close taking pictures, you could fall right in.

Thirty minutes away is Seljalandsfoss, which you can walk underneath. Although I was geared up in a waterproof jacket, pants, and rain boots, my face got soaked and was a bit uncomfortable. This waterfall was not like the one you can walk under in North Carolina. It is a much steeper, longer, and dangerous walk. I was concerned about Issa slipping; joy and excitement came to him as we walked closer.

While I stood back cautiously, Issa boldly lifted his face to feel the mist. I learned something about us at that moment. We are often in different frames of thought, and it's the checks and balances that keep us going. When I am cautious, he is liberal and free. When he is weary, I encourage him. When I am down, he says the most observant and encouraging things. I made an educated prediction that this dynamic will take us far.

We stopped for food on the ride back to Reykjavik. The pizza there, dare I say, rivaled a Brooklyn slice, but we had to buy a whole pie because it is not Brooklyn. My clothes felt heavy and damp, killing the mood for lingering. I hit the road as soon as possible to see our new home for the night. We reached Reykjavik at 7:30 p.m., not leaving time for much. We managed to make it to the Perlan Dome. Since they closed at 9:30 p.m., the girl didn't charge us full price. Issa was able to see the man-made ice cave, which he loved. The Northern Lights exhibit was closed, which really annoyed us. We didn't see the real or fake lights Northern Lights.

We went home wearing matching Iceland shirts, and I finished the trip in a teal bob. There were lots of looks and smiles. The guy next to me on the plane chatted me up the entire flight. When we got off the plane, he told his friend he just met his wife. We exchanged Instagram handles, and I never heard from him again.

Issa and I had sore throats most of the trip. I think that Blue Lagoon without robes was a terrible idea. It felt like our throats were going to fall out. We survived by taking Tylenol, which only helped the pain but didn't remove it. He cried at least once on the trip because he was so miserable. That was my evidence that things can be great and horrible at the same time.

I had no voice once I returned home, and we rested every second we could. It was a long school and work week. I see why people take a day off when they return from vacation. I was fighting for my life, and they told me I did not sound enthusiastic. I said, "My voice is brought to you by Nyquil," and ended up having to leave early on my first day back.

I definitely had a pattern of running away from home and responsibilities. After seeing a bunch of cool places, I wanted to make my home more polished and designed. In a dream, it came to me to make Issa a music room to keep him motivated to continue with his musical studies. The theme would be guitars, and they would be everywhere. He was gifted a few guitars and didn't use them. They were crammed under his bed and would make perfect displays. I found a guitar my sister sketched years ago and one of Issa's drawings from when he was young. He drew himself slightly better than a stick man with locs holding a guitar. Something was still missing. I found a Fender rug online. I waited for it to arrive and decided not to do the transformation until I had everything.

The biggest Marvel movie of the year was coming out on November 11, *Black Panther: Wakanda Forever!* I was personally so hyped about it that I purchased group tickets for my Hair Therapy crew to ensure we had the best seats and threw a premovie party with tons of Wakanda decorations, black and silver spoons, and a popcorn table. Getting ready was chaotic because I hosted a fifty-fifth surprise party for my Aunty at The Ritz Carlton the night before. I was barely home in enough time to cook and decorate. SWG attended and met an extended group of my friends, a different set of friends from my birthday at Swingers. He came toward the end when it was pretty lively. We took group pictures, he had dinner, and it was time to go. He offered to take Issa and me to the theater.

Eighteen of us attended; Issa and I were front and center. The new Black Panther was skinny like me, and I loved it. Being a skinny woman in the Black community, all I hear are songs about being thick and jokes about how no one likes skinny strippers with Brazilian butt lifts. Ultimately, the message I have received is that skinny women are not attractive because they don't have a shape.

Beauty was not the focus of this superhero; I just loved that she was very slim, and that was OK. Finding out she was Guyanese was galvanizing. That is me on the screen. I was inspired. I sat there processing what the loss of a mother can do to even a superhero. Ironically, I didn't get emotional until the end of the film. "My Name is Prince T'Challa, Son of King T'Challa." I had a tear for that heart-stopping child and how he introduced himself. Reminded me of my Prince Issa. It was also remarkable that they used such a powerful and popular Haitian name, which indicated that even more Black representation was on the way.

Once we returned to my house, the high energy from the guests converted to a mellow vibe. SWG and Issa played for a while, and I eventually sent him to sleep because he could stay up all night. I offered to box the rest of the food because, as a vegan, I surely wouldn't eat the rest of the wings, etc. When I put the food away, he stood in the kitchen next to me, and that was the first time I felt his presence. I almost wanted to stop what I was doing and look at him. I didn't. I carried on with the wrapping and the boxing. Once it became late, the hug for going home was long—like long. I didn't mind it. Felt a little safe. It seemed like a moment where first kisses happen. I thought a little about it while I took off my makeup. Every day we spent together felt like friends. It always had the friend feeling, but that day, it felt like a crush. But who has the crush? Does he like me, and do I like him back? Or do I like him, and he likes me back? Someone likes someone.

Ding dong! Amazon. My rug arrived, and that vibrant color really brought my room idea together. First thing in the morning, I put everything together while Issa was sleeping. It was going to be a surprise for his guitar lesson anniversary (November 15) and outstanding winter chorus concert (November 18).

He smiled and jumped like a rock star. I played *Teen Spirit* by Nirvana since that was the song he was learning that week, and it was one of his favorite songs in general.

To escape my usual winter depression, I proposed to my sister that we go to Aruba for her birthday. At the time, she flew for free. She planned to leave LA for Aruba and for me to go from DC to Aruba. My cheap flight had two stops and long layovers.

The first stop was Charlotte, so I used that opportunity to connect with the lovely lady from my friend's fiftieth birthday party. Issa and I met her at a donut shop and from there, we went to dinner. Our kids had a chance to talk and meet for the first time. I thought turning a layover into a play date was one of the coolest things I have ever come up with as a mom. We hung out with them until it was time to catch our second leg to LaGuardia Airport.

When we arrived at LaGuardia, it was late, and barely anyone was there. All the stores were closed.

The security guard said, "You have the option to be locked in the airport or outside." I chose in. Issa could not fathom that we would be hanging out in the airport from 10 p.m. to 6 a.m. We found a soft couch and caught our z's. I felt like a rag doll when I woke up, confused about where I was and what I was doing. I was eager to get on the plane. Once we arrived, the TSA officer insisted I put my carry-on in a bin that was barely bigger than my bag, and I ended up breaking a nail taking it out. Breaking a nail before even getting to your vacation destination is enough to choke a bitch. In lieu, I cut my eyes at her. The other question I had to ask myself is, if Miss Vickie had done my nails, would they have been strong enough not to break? I knew the answer was yes. Lesson learned.

Ninety-six degrees slapped me in my face and almost melted my North Face off. I liked it. I'm hot in December! What made this trip special was my sister's paternal ties to Aruba. We visited where her dad grew up and explored the less touristy side of the island. As usual, I spent hours mapping things out—every meal and three hotels. A new one every night. The Courtyard Marriott had the biggest and best pool. The Eagle Resort had a human-size checkerboard that Issa and his aunty enjoyed.

The trip's highlight was our stay at The Boardwalk Boutique Hotel and the vegan spread made special for my sister by Chef Djuric at The Ritz Carton. The Boardwalk Boutique Hotel is on a coconut plantation. The pool had no open or close time, so while hanging out there at night, I spoke to SWG. He looked like he was going out; we talked for a little bit, and I was happy about that. I liked the convenience of the Boardwalk beach. Guests received waiter service on the beach from the Ritz Carlton, and we took full advantage of that. There was a walk-up smoothie shack on the property. I love smoothies!!

The most impressive thing about Boardwalk is the atmosphere. There are coconut trees *everywhere*. It felt like you were in the jungle. The rooms are themed after little houses to make you feel like you live there, and each room comes with a grill. It is truly a dream. The textures and color scheme were refreshing—light pinks, white, teal, pops of yellow. The bathroom had a window that opened, and I heard birds chirping while I showered. I felt like I was on a retreat. I woke up early to record videos outside.

I grabbed my tripod and cutest Fenty Beauty set, and I had a ton of fun in the sun. I sported black braids with pink highlights in a bun. "Anti-hero" by Taylor Swift played in a loop in my head. That was going to be the song I used for my IG reels. I was in heaven out there frolicking. People were probably looking out of their casitas, wondering what I was doing and why I chose such an open area to do it. I wanted to show my environment and the greenery; I was really feeling it. There was a hammock on the porch, and when I wasn't snapping away, I was swinging there.

The unimaginable happened when we went to visit Baby Beach. I *relaxed*. I know; I wasn't expecting it either. Knowing my time was limited and unclear when I would return, there was pressure while on vacation. Trying to make it to all the places on my list, getting up early to put on makeup so my pictures looked great. The food was great and the pictures were perfect, but I was far from relaxed. I made a conscious decision to put my phone down. I had more than enough pics for the day.

I went far out in the water with my son to relax. Baby Beach is known for its low tides, and we were able to go further than we could at other beaches. I closed my eyes. I thought about the previous Decembers when I didn't have the resources to be anywhere but in my room. I thought about when I was a child, and my dad used to send me to Tobago for the summers. Being at the beach every other day used to be a regular part of life and how much times have changed. My Dad must have loved me to invest in me and expose me to more than Brooklyn, and now I was passing on the experience of traveling to Issa.

I also took a second to think of nothing and listen to the ocean and people around me. I felt my heart rate slow down. Real relaxation. I wish I could put that feeling in a bottle. Now I associate Aruba with letting my hair down. Our last dinner was at Ike's Bistro, which was scrumptious. I wasn't expecting to have my socks blown off. The food was melting in my mouth. The pool was glowing blue, and a man was playing the saxophone. The atmosphere was perfect.

    I came back ready for the rest of December. Straight back into the routine of studying math and science every day for at least two hours with Issa. Perimeter, area, volume, earthquakes, and volcanoes. Writing long letters to teachers to make sure assignments were turned in. I went back to the gym to work on my belly for the millionth time and attempted to keep my endorphins going.

    It was almost SWG's birthday, and this year, I kept it simple with dinner and a movie. He was dressed up for real and so was I. The theater was new and the first experience for us both. We went to see *Violent Night*. It was absolutely ridiculous and very violent. I don't give major gifts to men, so I got a card and a tiny bottle of Macallan. It was freezing that night, brutally cold. Luckily, he was heading on a guy's trip to tropical weather for his actual birthday. While he was there, he sent me a picture of my book. He was reading *Beautiful Reject* on vacation. I thought that was cool. I never read on vacation; I consider that work, but I know some people find it relaxing.

    January. I have loved calendars since I was a child. I liked writing down whatever took place that day in each box. Because I was always looking at the calendar and doodling in the calendar, I became very good at remembering dates. Now that I'm an adult, I use my calendar to write down everything for myself and my son. Once those dates were squared away, I started working on invites. I like to let people know very far in advance if I can make it to their birthday. I see an invitation to a birthday as something very special because it's the day someone came to Earth, and that's remarkable.

This year, I had my eyes set on a Passion Planner. My sister had given me a chic one the year before, and I liked the stickers and the structure. It was black with black and gold tabs and a lime green string bookmark. I was a little intimidated by the homework in front of the book and admittedly did not finish the work until around the end of the year.

One of my goals for January was to roll out a Hair Therapy University page to start a women's support group. My first idea was to teach finance since many New Year's resolutions were about financial achievements and physical fitness. I had the perfect teacher for the job, Dr. Rufaro. She taught a finance 101 course that was broken into three different sessions, each one more informative than the next. I was very proud of her presentation and grateful to have someone who invested their free time to teaching the community. I never got around to doing all of the advanced steps of the financial planning course, but I did learn to be responsible and stay current with all bills. A significant improvement from recent years. I loved that there was a financial health quiz in the presentation.

Things were changing with SWG and me. We texted a ton during the day. We spoke every night on FaceTime. He came to one of Issa's chorus concerts. The most notable change is that we stopped watching TV downstairs and started watching it on the floor in my room. We were not physical, and we never spoke about liking each other. A defining moment was when he called and said, "I know I said I would watch *Wednesday* with you, but I am headed down south in the morning. Could I stay with you and leaving the morning?"

I jumped up like, omg, it's happening; we are about to be on some other shit after today. I said, "Are we sleeping together or apart?" He laughed and told me he would see me later. I was serious, but since he didn't answer, I made the guest room so he could have his own space like a regular visitor.

Supposedly, he had injured himself, and I told him I would massage him whenever I saw him, since he did one for me when I almost broke my back training with him. The major difference is that my rub was in public. He used tiger oil on my lower back on the right; it was damn near lifesaving. I don't know what I was trying to prove by showing up for the workout, knowing I was in bad shape.

Fast forward to the present. We watched *Shot Gun Wedding,* and he paused it, inquiring about the massage. We head to the guest room. I lit a candle and found some music; I felt some nerves. *Under the Influence* by Chris Browne is not spa music, so we started in the danger zone.

I did a pretty professional job, in my opinion. I asked if there was anywhere else that needed rubbing. He said, "My chest if you are comfortable." Now I am in trouble for sure. He faced me and I straddled him. He said, "Your turn," and I think I turned red. I had to catch myself. I washed my face, I brushed my teeth, and I had a choice—go to my room or the guest room. I said, "You want me to sleep with you?" He said, "Do you want to sleep with me?" and I laid down.

It wasn't many rubs before his lips touched mine. I had an explosion of thoughts. Mainly OMG, OMG, OMG. Rubbing his hair, touching him felt foreign to me. He rubbed on me for hours. I could not fall sleep with all the caressing, and it felt really good. He was touching everything, and I let him. Like a high school girl, I was moaning and groaning over his fingers until I orgasmed on them. Although the moment was enticing, I knew I wasn't ready for sex. The equivalent of being fingered would be being jerked off. I blew right past that logic and kissed his head with my lips. It wasn't long until he orgasmed too. This time, when I got back in bed, all the rubbing stopped. He slept with his back to me. A foreshadowing of what was to come.

In the morning, he left to go down south, and my phone was dry. I was the one who asked if he made it to his destination. I was already feeling off. The next time we spoke, he did not look happy. I asked him what was going on, and he revealed that he was struggling with feelings for his ex. My head spun around.

"Your ex! Are you serious? Did you know you liked your ex before you asked to stay at my house?" I was an option. Ugh. Instant regret surged through me.

Thoughts: *You stupid bitch; you fell for the okie dokie.* That man did not establish a formal dating system with you. We did not discuss any intention. I partially caved in our first intimate moment together, and now he is done with me. He was here because I had no boundaries and was too damn friendly. He wasn't looking for a lover or a wife in me. Come on bitch, you wrote about this on page 13, Fantasy Theory. "Some encounters will leave you chewed up and spit out. The outcome is usually favorable when you are not prey. In your female fantasy, if you are the lioness, and in his fantasy, you are the zebra—well, you're gonna die!" This lesson was tough; just because I have been doing well for a while does not mean I can't fuck up. Ignoring the flags, ignoring my gut, and outcomes from prior mistakes will lead you back to square one.

That was the beginning of a bunch of text messages about what he didn't intend to do. I didn't intend this, and I didn't intend that. I was so fucking mad. I said, "So you read my book, watched my life, saw my weak spot, and tested me out for fun."

I cried for days. I could not believe that after four years and four months of minding my fucking business, I risked it all for a chump with no plan for me or my kid. He barely called me. We barely spoke. Whenever we did talk, it was long text messages overexplaining how he sees me as a friend and why I think he is an asshole. I crashed the fuck out multiple times. January was miserable. I thought about how happy I was dancing in the sun in Aruba. I missed her. I missed that happy, happy me. I was so unhappy with myself, and the rate at which I was discarded was so alarmingly fast. It made me question everything.

CHAPTER 6

JANUARY 27, 2023 - SEPTEMBER 27, 2023
CRASH OUT, THEN HEAL
(EIGHT MONTHS)

We still followed each other on Instagram, and the amount of subposting I did was embarrassing. He had apologized multiple times via text, but I was still mad. The texts were all the same. "Never meant to hurt you; I just want my friend back. You just wanted to get to know me. I am not sure what the disconnect is." Every single variation of how you could say the same exact shit, he said it.

I was hoping for, "I really fucked up. I would like to do this the correct way. You have nothing to worry about. I shut that shit with my ex down." I didn't work through all my feelings, but I knew I would not go back to friendship like nothing happened. From my perspective, that's how men get the best of both worlds. They get a little taste of you, keep you around, and still be with who they want. I gained too much experience with that in the past. It never gets better, and it is best to leave. Our shit just started a few days ago, and it was already ending, and I hated that. When he came back in town, he brought me some cookies that I asked for before he left, and shit was so dry. He was very awkward, and so was I.

February 6. I shared with my therapist that my chest was hurting, and she prescribed me a day off. I had been seeing her for a while, and this was the first time she had ever suggested time off. I did not question it. I obliged. I spent the day receiving an emergency service from One with Ebony, my long-time yoga instructor/masseuse. I had a Thai bodywork massage. It gave temporary relief, and the feeling came back.

My therapist always encouraged me to write down my feelings when I am feeling bad, whether its late night thoughts or issues that arise when we are not scheduled to meet. After I wrote my thoughts, if I didn't feel any better, I'd share those thoughts with her in my next session, and we would work through it. This is one of the letters I wrote to her after my day off.
Letter to My Therapist 2/10/24

> Dr. Crosby,
> I wish I had happier things to write to you. This week, my efforts were so high, and the results were so low.
>
> My chest continued to hurt most of the week. On my day off, I didn't go to the spa; I laid like a rock for eight hours. During the day off, SWG texted; he was worried and sorry, and I told him he was absolved and it's too late to worry about me.
>
> Wednesday, I got a bodywork Thai massage from a healer I trust. I cried through the whole thing. When I was there, I felt myself sinking into the ground when she said, "Feel your body sink." I felt I was lowered like a casket. Then I rose back up by the end and awoke.
>
> She said my mom was present and gave me an assignment to sit in front of a mirror each day for ten minutes, be still and accept myself, and wear a color from the chakra chart, starting with red (the root).

I felt renewed for an hour, and then my chest started hurting again. I hated seeing his face, and I hated the absence.

Wednesday evening, I hosted a stress and anger session, and I wasn't my usual self, but it was still very good for the participants.

In the past, I was speaking as a person who was past many obstacles, but this week, I felt like a crackhead trying to help other crackheads.

My son came into the room before the session and told me he doesn't want to grow up and life isn't what he thought it would be. He told me he doesn't want this life; he wants a new one because this one is ruined.

He cried, and I tried to assure him he was amazing. He said he didn't want to have ADHD and grow up to be a weirdo. I cried with him and felt so sad. I learned that he processes emotions like me. Harsh and heavy. It made me sad.

After drying his tears, I gave him the book and new Hot Wheels and told him how much I loved him and so did other people. It cheered him up.

When all the activity cleared out, I lay in bed alone and felt horrible.

Then I stayed up until 3 a.m. communicating with designers about my book. I haven't had any excitement about the book. As I plan for the release party and everything is coming together, I'm getting sadder and sadder.

As I post on Instagram, many people have been reaching out. Other women in pain or who want to speak about anger. I even connected with a friend whose dad died and her boyfriend broke up with her.

I do not want to be this person. I don't want to be hurt to be inspired to create and connect with the world. Like Issa, I am starting to resent life and what fuels most of my creative process.

I have been fighting for my life, but mentally, I don't want to do anymore. I'm soooo tired, and if I'm going to have a loveless life where no help is coming, I prefer to die today than drag it on. Having a son is the only reason I haven't jumped off the Woodrow Wilson. He is literally the only thing keeping me blinking.

I only see my potential future as my past patterns in the past seven years. More projects and isolation. . .or projects and heartbreak. I can't see projects and love and support; it is hard to imagine because I haven't seen it in so long.

Men are coming to me to comfort them and running off to marry and chase other people down; there is nothing I can do about it but be alone forever to protect myself, and that's so depressing.

I love my son, but even he feels the emptiness of this house and no one giving a fuck about us enough to love us as the primary people in their lives. They want to drive by and check-in but not live life with us. It's breaking us both. We both feel it, nonspecial enough, oddballs out, passed up.

When we make a big deal of ourselves, it presents well, but if we don't put on a show and show what we have, no one will give a fuck. Like if I never made shit, I was just a bitch that works, and he was a talentless kid. I can only imagine what that would be like.

I didn't see this coming, but now that I'm here, I feel too weak to fight. I'm so tired. My spirit hurts. I miss who I was before this because I thought I was actually making progress, and I was hopeful; I was annoyed but optimistic. Weary but determined. Now I'm like, fuck! I just got dealt a hand with no spades. Some people have partners and no talent; that's their cards. Mine is this a life full of everything but someone for me.

I wasn't speaking to SWG. Valentine's Day came and went without a word. In his absence, there was a guest appearance from Mr. Teenage Crush, and he was still fine as fuck. He saw my sexy *Beautiful Reject Coloring Book* promo photos on Facebook and said he had a gift for me and would bring it by. When he arrived, we talked a bit, I looked into his multidimensional eyes, listened to his deep voice and faint northern accent, but I held it together. At the moment, I felt proud of myself for not being at home withering away from my missteps with SWG. What sucked is my Teenage Crush still didn't really like me. He really is down to fuck, but he doesn't have a romantic bone in his body for me.

I better hold onto that kiss from tenth grade because I am never ever getting another one. That's just one of my rules. I'm never having sex voluntarily with a man that doesn't kiss me. That would make me feel like a blow-up doll. We kept it light and cute, nothing dramatic. When I told him I had been celibate for some time, he said, "Oh hell, no, that's a curse." I think a curse is a bit harsh. I could tell he was in OG player mode. He was transparent (after I asked, of course) that his heart belonged to his ex. I was the hospital for broken-hearted men. I enjoyed my last minutes of looking at his face and I still have the bottle of wine he brought me. That was hard because he was *fine*! Ugh. I am a walking test/lesson magnet.

February 17. I prepared for my book release party for *Beautiful Reject: The Coloring Book, Cognitive Distortions*. I received all of my beauty services on that day because I wanted to look fresh, and I didn't want my look leaked. I had very long dark red braids. A black strapless dress with a tutu on the bottom. Chrome red toes and red chrome stiletto nails. Next, I was off to get my neck and chest adorned with henna.

As I lay there with my eyes closed, I listened to the rapturous and soft voice of my henna lady, A. Ryze, as she spoke to her children. She sounded so calm and sweet. I was hoping she wasn't on drugs. I asked her if she was always that way and she replied, "No." She said she had some shadow work done by a woman named Rita. She had some tough times; she was hearing voices, and Miss Rita got to the bottom of it. Her husband and children noticed a big difference in her and her life has been better ever since. This was the first time I heard the term "shadow work." I wasn't sure what she was talking about. If there was ever a chance for me to sound so angelic while speaking to Issa, I wanted to try. She sent me Rita's information, and I reached out on Instagram.

That evening, I worked on some last-minute touches to the house as I waited for guests to arrive. I converted the entire house into a white and red theme. White tablecloths, red roses, and black chairs. A trusted chef catered the food, and I knew that everyone who could make it would love it. I had live music by a saxophone player, which was a surprise for the guests and a first-time hosting effort for me. It was a great touch, but all that jazz made me miss my dad. I called Dad on FaceTime so he could hear the tunes for a bit. I was let down when I learned my cousin who illustrated the book was not coming. I had a custom hoodie made for her, and collectively as a family, had bought her a ton of red roses to celebrate.

Toward the end of the night, I started to feel a little down. SWG didn't call and he didn't come. I just thought he would come or say good luck. I FaceTimed him and just blinked in his face. Eventually, I spoke, "You didn't come, wow." He said something about his car being broken the past few days and I listened. When we hung up, I was bothered. He was always around and now he wasn't.

I told him I had something for him, and I took food from the party. That's usually an end-of-night thing. I had never been to where he lived. That is also crazy. We spoke in the car a little, but it seemed the nicer I was being, the more distant and odder he was. I wanted to be enraged, but the lover in me was hurt. I could feel that I had no one. It really sucked that he treated me nicely like a plutonic girlfriend for two years, and since our intimate moment, things have been raggedy. All the shit a girl does not want.

My emotions were twirling around. No matter what he said, I was mad, and I wanted to go back to the phone call and say, "No." Undo the night and undo the pain. Also, the rejection fucked with me. Playing with me and not really wanting me was the trauma that made me quit intimacy, and I had picked right back up where I left off. I really thought I would break the seal of solitude with my next partner. I felt like a failure.

Another challenging thing was Issa asking about him.

"Where is he, Mom? I am going to call him." Issa FaceTimed and asked, "Why don't you come over anymore?"

He told Issa he was sorry, and they both had tears in their eyes! What the fuck! I did not know that my kid had these emotions about him. The Worst Mom on Earth award goes to me! He told Issa he could call him anytime, and now I felt like I was keeping them apart. Issa had already lost so much. I really didn't want to bring additional heartache to my baby. After this call, I agreed that he could still attend Issa's concerts so they could maintain contact. It wasn't the same as him being there every week, but it was something. We were never affectionate in front of Issa, so I was curious about his outlook and attachment to SWG.

I asked Issa what was going on. He said, "Well, Mom, I thought that you loved each other because you watched movies together and you love movies. You don't seem to watch them with anyone else. Also, I think he looks like me. Sometimes it is like looking at myself because he is silly like me too."

I was speechless. Kids are so observant. Proximity and consistently being around was enough for my son to see our friendship as a relationship. Now the friendship is a failed situationship. I promised myself not to let it happen again. I don't want anyone regularly coming over, even friends. This awareness had me in a weird place. I wanted to push SWG away because he caused pain and keep him around because he brought us comfort and familiarity. We had many routines together. My workdays changed, my weekends changed, my bedtime conversations changed. I was running hot and cold on a merry-go-round, and it showed.

My therapist observed my changed behavior and emotional letter and recommended that I see a woman named Dahlia. March 3 was the first day that I reached out to Dahlia. On our first conversation, I spoke a mile a minute, going on and on about my recent experience and how I felt used and stupid. She calmly said she would put something together for me based on what she heard. She had me at the headers. Past, Present, Future. All things I needed help with.

Past Session 1 (March 18th at 8:30am)	Present Session 2 (April 1st at 8:30am)	Future Session 3 (April 15th at 8:30am)
Modalities applied: Reiki, Pranashakthi, Sound healing, crystal healing, plant healing, energy body-field-channel recalibration, Akashic records healing, Ancestor healing.	Modalities applied: Reiki, Pranashakthi, Sound healing, crystal healing, energy body-field-channel recalibration, Akashic records healing, Ancestor healing.	Modalities applied: Reiki, Pranashakthi, Sound healing, crystal healing, energy body-field-channel recalibration, Akashic records healing, Ancestor Healing.
- Rebuilding the body and energy field from trauma the began in 2012 and then again in 2018. - Creating a safe space to resolve unhealed trauma.	- Introduction to your path in this life and how to apply your purpose in every situation you find yourself in.	- Shamanic journey to your future self on your current path.
- Soul Retrieval and extraction needed for trauma nestled in between muscles and within the cells. - A Limpia will be used to address family curses and trauma handed down.	- Bringing forward your gifts and how to use them. - Awakening how trust shows up in your energy/body.	- Getting clear on anything you with to manifest moving forward.
- Plant medicines and teas will be provided that support the healing and opening of the heart. - Additional tea will be left to continue the healing process after the session is over.	- Continued fascial release work will be used to bring you into the present moment and introduce you to who you have become at this stage.	Any activations that your soul calls in the will draw you closer to the highest version of who you can be in this life.
Breathwork	Breathwork	Breathwork
- Movement is necessary to wake up the forgotten parts of the self. - Embodiment movement will be used to reconnect the mind with the body and soul for a clearer pathway forward.	- A biomat and healing crystals will be brought in to support physical healing and relaxation.	- A biomat and healing crystals will be brought in to support physical healing and relaxation.
- A biomat and healing crystals will be brought in to support physical healing relaxation.	- 2 weeks of work (mantras, journaling, etc.) will be assigned and you will receive 2 check-ins during that time	- 2 weeks of work (mantras, journaling, etc.) will be assigned and you will receive 2 check-ins during that time
- 2 weeks of work (mantras, journaling, etc.) will be assigned and you will receive 2 check-ins during that time		

Dahlia is a Transcendental Counselor, priestess in the Order of Melchizedek, Crystal Intuitive and Specialist, Multiple Certified Reiki Master/Teacher, Pranashakthi Master/Teacher, and Soul Realignment Practitioner.

March17. SWG and I had a sit-down at a local bar and talked about what he had been doing lately. We were not talking, but he reached out because it was part of our routine. If we had a work meeting while we were already out, we would go out. It was clear we had some attachment issues because I was hoping he would call. I told him I was going to Virginia Beach a while back, and he said, "Oh, cool, I could meet you there." Now we were talking about whether to make dinner reservations on the beach trip. If things were not a mess, thinking about that would be exciting. We were in a fake break-up from our fake relationship, planning a fake family vacation. We were both fucking delusional, and I knew that. I wasn't ready to let go.

Dahlia

On March 18, when I opened the door, my eyes stared back at me through Dahlia. She was in white and I was in black. I knew that I met my match, not that I would ever challenge her. I just knew she was a real one. She asked me where I would like to be, and I said my room. She took some things upstairs and started setting up. She had some tea for me and selected my Mickey Mouse cup from the cabinet.

The first exercise included writing a letter and burning it. The other exercises took up to three hours. I released so much pain and tension in my body with this session. The experience was very sacred, thought-provoking, and mind-moving. I did simple things, such as close my eyes and lay on an amethyst mat, and I did complex things, which tested my discipline and the strength of my breaths. Generally, these sessions can take anywhere from one-and-a-half to two hours. My session took longer because I was carrying all sorts of stuff. I lost all sense of time and three hours felt like five minutes. When my session was over, I told Dahlia they were coming, even though I didn't know what that meant. The doorbell rang. It was my brother. I slept for several hours after my first session.

The most phenomenal thing about Dahlia was her detailed readings and soul retrieval capabilities. The readings were written out the day before and given to me to read as she set up for the session. The soul retrieval is item one of thirteen on the session summary worksheet.

The headers on my two-page reading were:
- The situation
- Being impacted by
- Below the surface/the subconscious mind
- What you have come through/things coming up from the past to be healed
- Should things continue as is, what could you expect
- The near future
- Where you find yourself
- Your surrounding/environment
- Fear
- Outcome

The reading was so in-depth. I felt complimented and, other times, insulted. Each header was followed by a paragraph of writing specifically for me. For example, an uplifting line in the March 18 reading was, "A project you have been nurturing will begin to come to fruition. This is a great time for travel as well. Within your inner realms, you will begin to experience more spiritual growth and change your belief system, which ultimately leads to more fulfillment. Money flows, connections are harmonious, and you may feel inspired to make improvements to your home." This sounded promising and accurate. It was palatable.

A portion of the reading made me want to put the paper down. "You may be feeling alone and unsupported. This is adding to physical stress in your body and could potentially lead to illness if it continues. The energy of isolation stems from your attitude/perception of what's happening around you rather than people truly not being supportive of you. Contributing to this feeling of aloneness is an avoidance of asking for help."

Wait a damn minute! It was getting too personal. It went on to say, "It may feel tempting to hold on to stubbornness and feel like you've seen it all before, and that feeling that others may not truly want to help or assist, but you are energetically in a time where you are attracting more aligned people and situations in your life. What is available to you at this time will be dependent on what and who you allow to be a part of your life. It will also depend on when you let your guard down and take time to accept people as they are without trying to draw out the best version of them." I was exposed.

I would like to take a moment to note that incredible recordkeeping and digital archiving are how I have been able to share this story. I am sorting through my past one moment at a time. Currently, as my fingers stroke my MacBook Pro, I've been shown that sometimes the messages are there, and I miss them. As I reread this reading from March 18 in the section headed, What you've come through; things coming up from the past, reads: "Self-expression was the guiding force, and you worked with your charm and enthusiasm to create change for yourself and others. That version of you is being called forward to reconnect with you to accomplish your goals and desires at this time period; you may find that merging with this previous version of you takes a little more work than you anticipated, but it will be worth the adventure. This version of you was able to *channel and automatic write*. Practicing those two intuitive abilities would help to bring some wholeness back into your life."

Channel and automatic write? I overlooked that in 2023. What does that mean exactly? I took a break to research, and these were my findings. "The basic process for working with automatic writing is simple: The aim is to relax into a very deep state of relaxation and then allow your mind to answer questions effortlessly and naturally." The process is asking yourself a question and writing everything that comes to you once you do. Read the writing and sift out received messages. They describe automatic writing as a powerful technique to channel your subconscious mind and connect with a higher source of inspiration, creativity, and insight.

This was so important for me to see because "writing to reality," which is what I called it before discovering the coined term, is something that I have noticed and been doing throughout my life. I have even saved some of the lists that I have written in the past because when I wrote them, I was in a seemingly hopeless situation; once I completed the list, my life was changed for the better.

I was always so intrigued by this and quietly proud of it. What happens when we stop doing things that have worked for us and do not replace them with a better system? Times that I didn't take the time to center myself and write caused me to stay in longer bouts of depression, and I see that now. My need to grab a pencil and map things out is not an odd quirk; it's a part of my superpower. It is an instrument. I observed how readings integrate what has happened and is around you with various ways of showing us how my accountability and thought processing affect the outcome of my life.

During soul retrieval, numbers are called, representing your age when that piece of your soul left. When she called those numbers, my eyes would open. I knew exactly what she was speaking about. Imagine something bothers you so much when it happens to you that a piece of your soul leaves. Are you really forty if the four-year-old version of you just leaves and doesn't come back?

The numbers that came up in session one were four, twenty-nine, and thirty-five. These pieces of my soul are the ages that came back to me in session one. Four is the age at which my mom left me with my dad. She knocked on the door and said, "You take her," and he did. I didn't see her much until I was about seven years old. Twenty-nine was the age I delivered Issa, and thirty-five, my age when my mother passed. My homework was to go to the mirror for seven days, look myself in the eye, and say, "I love you and welcome home." Additionally, do things that I enjoyed at those ages.

Other sections on the session summary sheet were:

- Spirit animal messenger
- Karmic energy bodies/points (areas that may be impacted initially or chronically)
- Sage bath assessment
- Congested areas of energy noted intuitively
- Limpia cleansing
- Congested areas of energy noted by the limpia process
- Chakra limitations
- Hex crossings (instances of unintentional negative energy sent your way)
- Curses (instances of intentional negative energy sent your way)
- Unresolved trauma formations energetic appearance/ energy field appearance
- Entities/attachments/sentinels
- Spirit guides/ancestors present

The most shocking numbers were hexes, too many to count, curses at twelve, and the most comforting spirit guides/ancestors present hundreds. Dahlia and I completed many different exercises. It was a spiritual workout plan. Some components were unearthly and describing them would be a grave injustice.

Other paperwork that accompanied my initial session was a six-page astrology and healing report. The report came from a trusted astrologer of Dahlia. In essence, it's another person's perspective of me that I haven't even met. I didn't expect that. Imagine reading a complete book report about yourself. Something I found interesting was the summary of Sun, Moon, Rising, Mercury, Venus, Mars, Jupiter, Uranus, Neptune, Saturn, Pluto, Lilith, and North Node. I've only heard others discuss the moon and rising in general conversation. Last, the "Journal Prompts and Questions to Ponder" page. It had a list of prompts to be completed once a day. Below the prompts are recommended exercises for practicing presence and building trust.

On March 22, Issa had a bass concert, and SWG came to that. I was already there in the front row, and he texted me, "Twinkle, Twinkle," which was the song that was playing. I looked up and saw him. This was a pyramid concert with a middle school, and it included lots of kids. Issa was in fifth grade, so it was a big deal for him to participate with a larger crowd and bigger kids. Issa's sister and her mom were there also. We all took pictures and gave Issa his congrats and SWG went straight home after.

Soon after, we squeezed in a movie-turned-sleepover before I went to California to support my sister's surgery. I didn't make it until the day after her surgery because I refused to miss

Issa's concert. I would be away from home from March 24 to 29. On the way to Cali, my connecting flight was delayed, and I ended up staying in Boston. SWG and I spoke on the phone, and he had a questionable look. He said that I was mushy and he wasn't used to that. Again, I blinked. I told him, "You can be free of me." I went to bed angry, confused, and frustrated, but sure I had had enough of him.

I carried my journal on this trip and was always writing and keeping up with my journal prompts for Dahlia. I wanted to do anything but text my feelings. I set up a reading with Talk to Tash, who I heard about on the radio. Trying to connect with Rita wasn't working; I tried on February 17 via the website and on February 24 on IG. I reached out to A. Ryze on February 25 and 27 to see if she could get through to her on my behalf. No luck. As I was rolling in my Uber from the airport to my sister's house, I received a message from Rita saying she was doing some spiritual work and was away for a while. We scheduled my reading for Saturday, March 25.

Rita

Rita did a prayer and got straight to it. She is a fifth-generation hoodoo practitioner. I was glad to have a pen and tried to write down everything she said. This was my first reading where the person was speaking to me in real-time. She covered so many things very quickly.

- My mother went through a lot as a child
- Expectations were placed on her that were not in alignment with her
- She spoke about the explosive energy of my mothering
- My root chakra being missing
- Closeness with a narcissist and a womanizer

- My dreams trying to tell me stories that I could not grasp due to lack of balance
- My heart and roots not being on the same frequency
- My daydreaming and being on autopilot
- Seeking guidance that I would only be able to find through prayer
- Harvesting a dream I had in 2018 about creating an app
- Using technology to create things for Black people and other gifted people
- My spirit not feeling good here and spending lots of time transmuting
- Regression and going backward, standing on the cliff instead of jumping off of it
- Loving myself is the first template of how I want to be loved
- I spend no time by myself
- I need to learn to detach from Issa so we don't become codependent
- Plan a trip to Guyana to speak to an elder
- Block and remove men of the past from your social media
- Manipulation in my life is causing the yo-yo effect
- I have already dreamed my reality and future
- I am a starseed, light years ahead of my current time
- Write a letter to myself and burn it. Write a letter to my mother and burn it.

It was a lot to take in. I didn't know what to expect, and the reading made me think about many things. I wondered who the sheep in wolf's clothing was born between February 18 and 22? What is a starseed? Why do I transmute? How did she know about the app? I haven't thought about that app since 2018.

Hoodoo

Hoodoo is a tradition, a generational heirloom, that is simultaneously medicine, magic, and religion. Born on North American soil to African parents, hoodoo is a system of survival, adaptation, resistance, and reclamation. (hoodoosociety.com) The first written references to hoodoo appeared in 1849 in a Natchez, Mississippi newspaper. (wrldrels.org)

According to NPR, slave codes did not allow large gatherings of free or enslaved Blacks, and it was a crime for African Americans to practice traditions from Africa. As a result, some Hoodoo practices were hidden in African American churches, creating a unique brand of Christianity that fused African traditions that were called Afro-Christianity or African American Christianity. The Hoodoo religion during slavery included religious practices from various African cultural groups, including the Odinani religion of the Igbo people, the Yoruba and Vodun religions of the Fon and Ewe people, and a Bantu-Kongo tradition in Central Africa.

The United States is a vast land with varying ecologies. Regional Hoodoo is influenced by the African ethnicities brought to the area (often determined by skill) and local ecology. (hoodoosociety.com) Hoodoo doctors with a reputation for success invariably gained influence over those individuals who respected and often feared them. Most often, the reputed power of conjurers impacted individual bondsperson. Some, including antislavery activists Frederick Douglass and Henry Bibb. https://wrldrels.org/2020/05/04/hoodoo/

The visions they tried to depict in the movie *Harriet* were a cinematic take on her visions. The celebrated Harriet Tubman (1822-1913), one of the architects of networks that freed slaves (the Underground Railroad), was a conjuror, according to oral tradition. In those times, "It was called Conjure, Rootwork or Tricking. In the post-slavery era, the term Hoodoo was adopted."

The conjuror, male or female, was highly respected on the plantations. They cast spells for protection, vengeance, and love. They healed the sick with herbs (hence the name root worker). In other cases, they became the backbone of many slave rebellions. https://jamaica-gleaner.com/article/news/20181202/religion-culture-hoodoo-life-saving-magic-southern-slaves

Talk to Tash

My appointment was already on the books for Talk to Tash on Wednesday, March 29, and I was curious how her reading would compare to Rita's; would she say similar things or something completely different? I submitted two pictures prior to the thirty-minute session. I submitted one of Classic Man and one of SWG. This is what Talk to Tash had to say.

- Looking for love; focus on you right now
- Focus on Hair Therapy, grow and expand, find peace through a traveling network, and connect
- Envision what you want
- Everything is virtual in your life, and you are not connecting with others
- You need a healthy mix of virtual and in person

Her feedback on SWG: He is not ready to settle down. I am not the first woman he played with, and I won't be the last. He also dated women with kids in the past and created similar experiences for them as well.

Her feedback on Classic Man: He is just nosey and curious about what you are doing. He has not changed. He is exactly the same. If you re-engage, things will be no different than they were before.

I was also allowed to ask two questions. My first was, "Will the struggle with love ever end?" She said, "Yes. You will meet your partner through your work, Hair Therapy."

I asked, "Will my son be OK?" She said he would outgrow the issues he is currently having. He needed a mentor, a sport, track or soccer specifically, and that he would continue to be musically gifted. We both needed sleep and to meet new people.

I was defeated by her feedback overall. I was quiet the rest of the day and annoyed. I felt that my life required me to do too much before I was eligible for love while others were waking up and getting it. I didn't like being told to focus on myself because it seems like some cliché shit everyone says when you go through a breakup. I didn't like that the man of the past and the present meant nothing regarding my happy ending. I didn't like it.

After five days of quiet, SWG asked if he could pick me up from the airport when I returned. Of course, I said, "Yes." I have to be one of the only people who goes someplace to reset myself and comes crashing headfirst right back into it. I was really quiet in the car. He asked questions until he got me to open up a bit.

I told him it's not the best to be in a situation where you are trying to do things with me accidentally and not on purpose. That is a huge red flag. Acting like we are dating, then acting like we are friends, breaking up when we were not together, making up. It feels like you just want to casually go as far as you can, and I deserve better than that. I am resistant to making up because I know we will go right back to the great in-between. Even being here for me right now—it's 5 a.m. Who picks a girl up at 5 a.m. if they are not head over heels for her? The action makes it seem like you are really feeling me, but you're "friending" me to death. I expressed how much it sucked being on the other side. If I had known it would be miserable, I really would have stayed your friend; the treatment was way better. This was a calm conversation. I told him thank you, and he told me thank you. When I went inside, I continued to write in my journal, followed the prompts, and prepared for my next session with Dahlia.

Dahlia Session 2

April 1, 8:30 a.m. It was time for session two with Dahlia, and a new reading was in. This one-page summary spoke about me coming to terms with all that has happened. A wounded ego that controls my narrative will only distract and deter me from my deepest calling. It declared that it was time to let my light shine and bring my wisdom and learning into spaces where I can be seen, heard, and embraced.

The most prominent lines in the reading stated that I allowed relationships/connections to hold me hostage in the past. I've made myself a "good prisoner" of my circumstances and beliefs. My adaptability is a gift that has not been used for its highest potential. I hold the key to my cell and all the little things that have caused a buildup of frustration and annoyance. Once they are embraced as they do not require change from me, that will be the key to releasing myself. I will recognize the strength I built while I was in prison. I read that at least three times. I didn't see myself this way, but it did seem to be highly likely that I was living my life in a self-made prison.

It went on to outline that I am embarking on a new journey of love. Declared that real love is free to move and evolve. Healing my inner child will come to pass, and this healing will extend to my son. Be cautious of how I invest my time and energy. More than ever, light will be shown upon fake connections and commitments I have made. Decisions will have to be made about love on all levels—the love of family, friendships, my home, work, and life itself. I was asked to walk away from the past, and while it may feel like I have nothing, life will respond quickly and bring me into new spaces. Acceptance was key.

A new section was added that was not there before. Gifts and abilities. As I reread this section, it is like seeing it for the first time. This is why reflection is important.

Gifts and Abilities

- Automatic writing
- Clairvoyance
- Clairsentience
- Wayshower
- Alchemist
- The gift of authority (when speaking)

We already learned about automatic writing. I continued to seek the definitions of the other words listed.

Clairvoyance is the ability to communicate with dead people, predict future events, or know about things that you did not actually see happen or hear about. https://www.britannica.com/dictionary/clairvoyance

Clairsentience is a metaphysical sense that relates to recurring physical and emotional feelings. This is known as "clear feeling" and signifies Divine guidance. https://www.intuitivejournal.com/what-is-clairsentience/

Wayshower is an individual who has traversed the challenging terrain of self-discovery and has emerged with profound wisdom and insight. A Wayshower serves as a guiding light, illuminating the path for others who seek personal growth, healing, and spiritual awakening. https://consciousnessintervention.com/uncategorized/what-is-a-wayshower/

The definition of **alchemist** did not clarify anything. I had to dig deeper. "Spiritual alchemy is the art of inner transformation and liberation. Unlike its material counterpart, it focuses on the transmutation of the soul rather than physical elements. The spiritual alchemist seeks to refine their consciousness, purify their spirit, and ultimately achieve a state of enlightenment.

The journey of a **spiritual alchemist** is one of profound self-discovery and inner growth. It involves peeling away layers of conditioning, confronting deep-seated fears, and embracing the transformative power of consciousness." https://spiritualityessence.com/spiritual-meanings-of-alchemists

My soul retrieval number from session two was eleven. My chakra limitations and disconnections went down from five areas to two areas. Hexes/crossing reduced from too many to count to fifteen. Curses were reduced from twelve to three. Unresolved trauma formations were reduced from four to two. My spirit guide presence increased from hundreds to thousands. Thousands really made me smile (to think I was impressed with hundreds).

The handwritten bullet points Dahlia added to my summary worksheet were:

"You were seen in this lifetime as a child who had to steal food to eat. You continued to steal from one particular baker. One day, before you could steal from him, he offered you bread for free. You were suspicious but moved by his kindness. This thought taught you that you could receive from kind hearts and did not have to manipulate or take for fear of not having."

- You saw Egyptian themes
- You saw your son
- You heard Queen of Queens and Son of Sons
- You called for green or purple
- You saw yourself as an avatar

I saw a distinct memory, and I heard the rain and loud crashing thunder. The sound synchronized with my thoughts perfectly. I opened my eyes to discover that the rain and thunder were happening in real-time, and it wasn't a meditation soundtrack. I paused and said, "Am I Storm?" She moved to the next exercise. Dahlia was so mysterious, and I thought that was so fucking cool. Toward the end of this session, my brother arrived unannounced. I asked her, "What is going on?" She replied, "Healing extends."

April is for Issa 2023

What a powerful way to start off the month. I was feeling so much better. I could breathe without pain in my chest. I was looking forward to Issa's birthday, and I had a big trip planned to celebrate it.

Issa has dreamed of visiting Italy since learning about Venice from watching an episode of *Garfield*. This year, I learned of his interest in the Eiffel Tower after a school project he shared with me. I managed to squeeze a surprise within a surprise. He found out about Paris several days after the trip started. He cried tears of joy when we arrived in Paris, and that made my soul sing. I've never seen that type of tears from him before. Tears of Joy.

"Mom, I have dreamed about this my whole life. All of this just for me? I feel so special."

The plan was to arrive in Venice at 1:30 p.m., spend one night, at midday, take the bullet train to Milan (three hours), spend a night, take the bullet train to Paris (four hours), spend two nights. For the route back, take the train to Geneva, Switzerland (a small piece of Switzerland wedged between Italy and France; a common train change stop on rides back to Italy), spend one night. Then from Geneva back to Venice for two nights to relish in the canal vibes before leaving.

Venice planning was complex to navigate with many water routes. I was unsure how to make it to certain places until I arrived and was given additional assistance. I stayed somewhere easy to access from the airport by bus in Dorsoduro. At the end of the trip, I made the extra effort to stay deeper in Venice in San Marco to visit the shops.

What I planned and what happened were two different things. We got stuck in Milan and spent an extra night on the way to Paris. I could not catch a train to France due to a planned train strike I did not know about. I purchased a flight to Paris that morning, which was canceled later that evening. It took thirty days to get a refund.

This cancellation caused a delay and a domino effect for the rest of the trip. I missed some reservations entirely and was a day late for two reservations. With limited options for leaving Milan, I rented a car from SIXT and drove to Paris. I left around 3:30 p.m. and arrived at 3 a.m. After checking in, I drove to see the Tower immediately. There was no traffic, not one person on the street. It was our moment to have Paris to ourselves before the morning chaos began.

The travel time was twelve hours. While I was driving, SWG texted me to see how I was doing, and it was so hard trying not to respond, so I did but didn't say anything mushy. More just seeing how you are as a friend shit. I left to detox, and now I was thinking about him. I def thought that infrared photo at QC Termemilano would have him in a chokehold. Everyone else liked it, including him, but he talked about going one day with no mention of me.

After day two of the trip, I booked new reservations while missing out on the reservations I already paid for elsewhere. This was a complete waste of any savings and blew the budget planned for the trip. I had no travel insurance on the rooms and missed all the cancellation periods. No refunds were issued to me. Both Hotel Hoy and Hotel Bernina offered gracious special rates for the unplanned extension.

On the voyage back, we got stuck in Milan again because trains don't run late at night on Easter Monday, and we missed the last train out at 8:25 p.m. We spent an unplanned night in Milan. This was the most disastrous night of the trip.

The night in Milan was the most stressful of the trip. Driving back from France seemed to take forever. I almost always drive at night, but I wanted to see the fountain and catch the shops in Switzerland. We left Switzerland at noon. The day driving had us stuck in excessive traffic, and we didn't return the rental until 9 p.m. We took an Uber from the rental location to the train station. The rental place did not have twenty-four-hour personnel but gave us a gate code. It was a dark, isolated business park. The Uber arrived quickly, so I had no time to worry.

It cost $45, although the app quoted $30. At the station, we received confirmation that we had missed the last train back to Venice. Security gave us the option to stay with the police and sit on a bench from 11 p.m. until 5 a.m. or to get a hotel across the street because the station closes at 1 a.m.

The security guard recommended a place and told me to be careful crossing the street. The hotel was 650 feet away according to my GPS, and I still unknowingly missed a turn and walked too far up. Even though our luggage had wheels, it was cumbersome and loud. We passed four men smoking and my stomach sank. I felt odd. I asked Issa if he thought we would be

OK and he said, "No, we need an Uber." After just paying $50 to get to the station, I proceeded to walk.

A black Mercedes van passed me several times, first with a passenger, then perpendicular at the bottom of the street. Then, he was parked and smoked something that smelled like grapes. He looked into my eyes, and I looked down.

Seconds later, a man approached, saying, "My sister, I feel in my heart that man is following you and will steal your daughter. Let me help you; where do you want to go?"

I declined his help and he insisted I was in danger. I called the police; they put me on hold for a translator. I called back; the second person spoke enough English to ask where I was. I couldn't read the signs or pronounce my location with certainty.

I could see the van's headlights at the top of the block. This was now his third time circling the block. The man with the pink fanny pack claiming to have my safety as a priority said, "Don't go to the top of the block."

I felt tears in my eyes. My phone was at 10 percent. I called an Uber; it was four minutes away but taking forever. The van drove down the block and rolled down the window. It was a shiny black Mercedes, and the windows were pitch black. The driver said, "Would you like a ride?" I said very loudly, "No, thank you. No ride, no help."

I walked briskly to the top of the block. I saw a man and woman walking by and called out to them. "Excuse me; what is the number for 911 here if I need help?"

He said, "Don't talk to them; they are Italian. They do not care about you!"

The couple said, "We are not Italian!" got offended and walked away. I wanted to leave with them and hoped my question would alert them that I was in trouble, but that did not work.

I quickly requested a second Uber. The driver was one minute away. While we waited, the man with the fanny pack tried to take Issa's luggage twice, as I screamed, "Give it back!"

I called my Uber and asked him to please hurry. He said, "I am driving, ma'am; no talking and driving." He pulled up in a black Mercedes sedan, and I ran to the car, but not as quickly as the man who would not leave me alone.

The Uber driver was about to close his trunk and leave me, annoyed at whatever was being said to him in Italian. I said, "I am a US citizen." I showed him my passport and told him, "I must leave right now, please." I began to throw my luggage in the trunk when he re-opened it. He took it out and said, "Calm." I ran into the car and took Issa with me. The driver put my luggage in while screaming at the man with the pink fanny pack in Italian. He kept telling him he was calling the police and to "fuck off."

When we finally pulled away, I started crying and saying, "Thank you." He took me to the hotel I couldn't find, and it was two blocks behind us. Two blocks! The check-in process took forever, and the attendant asked for everything but a blood sample. Issa and I didn't take our clothes off; we were in shock. We FaceTimed family and friends to tell them of the experience until we were calm enough to go to sleep. I called SWG and told him I was almost stolen, and he looked a little too calm about it.

The hotel was extremely secure, so much so that we could not work the elevator in the morning without the access code and missed our train. Luckily, I paid an extra $9 for flexibility, and they moved us to the next train at 8:15 a.m.

This bullet train didn't go directly to the part of Venice I was trying to get to, known as the island. I barely got off at the correct stop in time. Thank goodness I did, or I would have ended up deep in another part of Italy.

We had to take a local train from Venezia Mestre by the airport to Venezia S. Lucia. Buying the tickets online on the platform was easier than getting one from the customer service desk. The line was out the door.

Now I'm running on fumes, trying to at least lay eyes on the hotel I was supposed to be in the night before and, at a minimum, get my son on a ferry so he can experience some type of boat. I felt like cattle packing onto the ferry, and it took a while to get to San Marco.

The walk to the hotel from the dock almost killed us—tons of steps—and the directions were a maze. When we arrived at the hotel, they revealed that there was no elevator! I wanted to pass out while a customer service representative was speaking. We took long showers and made the most of the six hours we had until it was time to leave for the airport.

While I was shopping for souvenirs, Issa spilled Gelato everywhere; his fingers were sticky, and his coat was a mess. I had to abandon gift hunting to get him cleaned up. The public bathroom cost $1.50 and smelled terrible. I decided to go back to the hotel. I still wish I could have made it to some of the cool T-shirt and bracelet shops. In a blink, it was 5:45 p.m., and the plane left at 8:30 p.m. I thought of the shlep we had getting to the hotel and kindly asked the concierge for a taxi boat.

He said, "They are quite expensive." I said, "Sir, I am asking you to call the boat, not how much it will cost."

We had to walk through a tunnel and a tiny pathway. The walk was very short compared to all we had been through. The sailor arrived a tiny bit late, which was a relief. We hoped we hadn't missed him since that was the theme of the day. He loaded the luggage and took my hand, and his hand touching mine was the best feeling. I could feel that a bit of fun was on the way. Once we got to the open water, the boat picked up speed, and my son's eyes lit up. There it was. Joy after trauma. This boat ride gave a new meaning to saving the best for last. Twenty-seven minutes and $150 later, we were at the airport, very much on time. We were greeted and told which counter to check-in. We were guided to the expedited family security line, boarding started extremely early, and, just like that, we were gone.

The layover in Istanbul was eight hours, and I wished I had booked the airport hotel in advance to be comfortable. The free sleeping area was packed, and the paid sleeping pods looked like something for quiet, relaxed adults, not Prince Issa. When it was finally time to board, Issa was about to cry when he overheard the man at the counter say we didn't have a window seat. The attendant empathetically changed our seats to the very first row. We had tons of legroom and a window seat. Issa turned the waterworks off, and I appreciated the upgrade.

When we landed nine hours later, police approached the plane looking for a passenger. I was convinced I was on a TV show and no longer in my real life. SWG did not offer to pick us up, so we Uber'd home. He told me that his aunt died the day I arrived, and he was not well. My body was weak, and I slept for days. The extra-long flight really took me out. When I felt better, I invited him for seafood and gave him a bulk beverage as an offering for the death in his family. I also got him a red shotglass from Switzerland.

During my trip to Italy, I learned to watch the current events of places I am headed, not just statistics on crime. My dad thought I was under a rock when I told him I did not know about the strikes. Also, to have a safe word for my kid in a tough situation, which means run. Make sure the phones are fully charged, and my kid has an Uber app with a form of payment downloaded to his phone and a credit card in the phone case. Make sure he has his passport in his jacket. If he has to run away, he has everything he needs on him. This is primarily when traveling with a lot of luggage and it is just the two of us. Issa said he wanted to run, but he was afraid to leave me. I wanted him to run, but I also knew he had nothing to help him survive.

Dahlia Session 3

April 14, 2023. SWG came over. It escapes me what we watched, but he stayed over. I got myself all healed up and went right back to the source of confusion and doubt. My healing session was at 8:30 a.m. It was 7:15 a.m., and this man was lying in my bed. I had a headache. I was doing this all wrong, and I knew it.

I reached out to Dahlia and confessed that SWG was with me, and I had a headache. She told me to pay attention to how my body was reacting to my choices. She came by and gave me a bracelet she restored for me. When I tried to reschedule, she said there was no need. Her parting gift was the written reading that was completed the night before. I felt horrible.

To make matters worse, the next day on FaceTime, SWG said he didn't feel anything the other night. The combination of missing my last healing session and getting played again was the complete opposite of self-love. I regressed in my thoughts of self-worth, and my head was filled with anger. I really was a sucker for punishment.

As I read through the updated energy, paragraph five stood out. "You are being cautioned that if you give up too easily on things that are positive, making progress in your life, you may find yourself ill and overly stressed. It will be important for you not to give up on your healing process in the next four weeks. Remain detached; be open to moving from fantasy into working on the details of the life you want."

I did not remain detached, and I definitely gave up. All that healing made me feel much better, and I took the strength and sanity I had gained from it and went right back to a situation that didn't serve me. I was giving CPR to a dead situation instead of calling a time of death. The weeks that followed had negative self-talk, empty feelings, and sad feelings. Even when we didn't speak and I was quiet. I wasn't proud of myself. I felt like I failed at healing.

SWG rejected commitment while "Checking in to see if I am OK." Isn't it supposed to be simple? If something feels bad, stop. What is my driving force for trying so hard? I wanted the intimacy to be meaningful. It was hard to accept that it wasn't. That physical affection didn't equate to deep emotional connection and commitment. I was trading small moments of comfort for weeks of confusion and doubt. Like paying $500 for a bag of chips. I love BBQ chips, but the price was too high. The cost of this was balance. I was very unbalanced. There was no rewind button, only an acceptance button.

Thoughts I still had in April:

- Why did he sleep in the bed with me if he had no feelings for me?
- Why am I so tired of self-care and the entire journey?
- Why do I feel like there's no point in living if I'm going to have a loveless life?
- What makes me go against my intuition?

Negative rumination was dominating. To show my state of mind, I compiled some of my texts. The roller coaster from reasonable to apologetic to blind rage. When someone says they are beside themselves, this is what they are talking about. I didn't even know I could get this mad anymore. I thought that ship sailed in February 2021. He and I were writing so much, saying the same shit in circles.

We shared some of the longest, dragged-out texts. These were some of mine.

Text 1 (4/21/23):

- Thank you for making the effort to connect, for apologizing, and recognizing my feelings yesterday
- Ultimately, I'm still unclear if you meant what you said and felt bad about how I reacted, or if you were trying to backtrack your words altogether after further thought.
- When you come back after I give up and leave you alone, I have no idea why you're back/which part of me you hope to reconnect with
- I am at a space where I am willing to let it all go in an effort to preserve my dignity and not become a yo-yo
- I am at a point in life where I want to figure it out together or walk away peacefully, but trying harder alone isn't an option
- I know there is a middle somewhere, but I have no idea how to obtain it or if I want it
- I think it's because I see the middle as purgatory most times; I seldom find joy in the land of in-between; not sure how everyone else does
- I am repairing and learning how to regulate my emotions every day
- My top goal in life right now is mastering the art of balance
- I've been trying to figure out what true self-love looks like; I was doing self-care often, but it has been brought

to my attention that is not self-love
- I support your interest in your own self-love discovery as well as therapy and hope you commit to both journeys
- I will not do anything to hinder your process of self-development
- I am not expecting anything from you at this time
- Please remove any perceived notation of pressure
- My expectations have changed as you have become more honest with me about your wants and capacity for processing me and life itself
- I am striving to become a better listener
- You are welcome to correct any takeaways I may have gotten wrong

My cumulative takeaways from your verbiage:

- ☐ You don't want a relationship with me or anyone at this time
- ☐ You are physically attracted to me
- ☐ You are not fully comfortable being intimate with me or telling me certain things, and you don't know why
- ☐ You think about sending me messages sometimes
- ☐ This situation is convoluted/no different than any other messy situation, and time may reveal something different than we see now, or maybe it's exactly what it looks like
- ☐ Work is taking a toll on you (it has been escalating in recent days)
- ☐ You are actively seeking therapy to release your thoughts in a safe place and beginning a self-love journey

My overarching key points I strived to convey:

- ☐ I prefer dating on purpose, not by accident
- ☐ I am not ready for sex, but I learned through our experience I am ready for some intimacy. I value G-rated

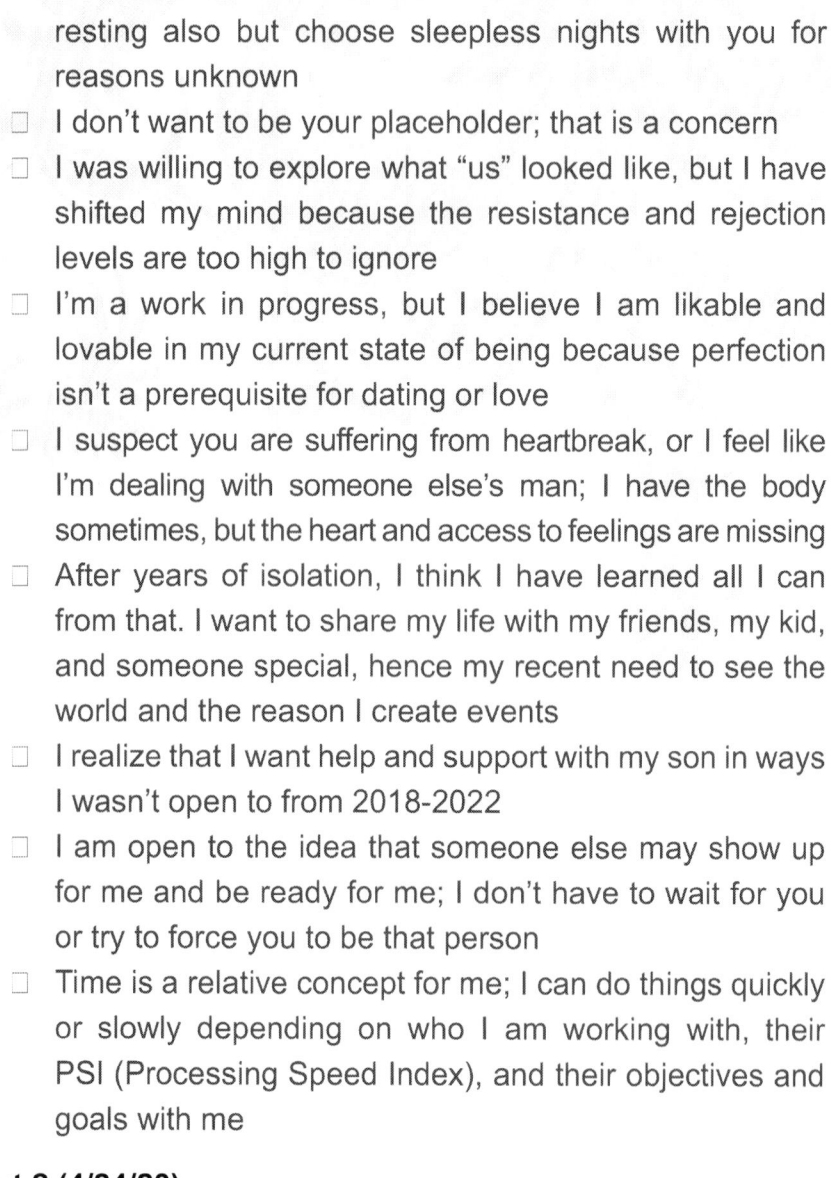

- resting also but choose sleepless nights with you for reasons unknown
- I don't want to be your placeholder; that is a concern
- I was willing to explore what "us" looked like, but I have shifted my mind because the resistance and rejection levels are too high to ignore
- I'm a work in progress, but I believe I am likable and lovable in my current state of being because perfection isn't a prerequisite for dating or love
- I suspect you are suffering from heartbreak, or I feel like I'm dealing with someone else's man; I have the body sometimes, but the heart and access to feelings are missing
- After years of isolation, I think I have learned all I can from that. I want to share my life with my friends, my kid, and someone special, hence my recent need to see the world and the reason I create events
- I realize that I want help and support with my son in ways I wasn't open to from 2018-2022
- I am open to the idea that someone else may show up for me and be ready for me; I don't have to wait for you or try to force you to be that person
- Time is a relative concept for me; I can do things quickly or slowly depending on who I am working with, their PSI (Processing Speed Index), and their objectives and goals with me

Text 2 (4/24/23):

And the apology in a week or a month. Keep it! Apologize to yourself and I'll do the same. You weren't feeling me since you fumbled trying to express it in Boston. What you meant to say was, I'm sorry, but I feel nothing for you even when you shower me with affection. I stepped off so smooth from that convo, you just had to drag me back in!

Anyway, I'm going back to September 19, 2020, the day before I met you. I'm no longer interested in "moving forward;" move me backward because I don't trust you, from the crown of your head to the soles of your feet. I don't get you, and I'm not about to die an emotional death trying to figure you out. Cause we all saw how figuring it out "together" worked out! That was some BS. Men in Black me, then Men in Black yourself, please! I'm light years away from whatever is going on in your mind, so it is not astonishing that your energy can't connect with mine. I'm not on your planet, possibly even galaxy. Before you even question why the rage, I always found it so corny that I had to approach you to learn about the "issues of the day" you had with me. It's fucking stupid. You always on some "I was about to tell you fucking BS."

Text 3 (4/24/23):

"I DON'T KNOW WHAT I WAS THINKING! Giving a basic-ass dude the opportunity to treat me like a worthless bitch. What's the point of healing then meeting men like you?! I'll never understand why I gotta be consistently fucking tested and tried instead of blessed with encounters that are healthy. The fucking smug, aloof look on your face when you say the most fucked up shit makes me want to knock your head straight off your neck!

While you have successfully destroyed any soft feelings I had left, you have also ignited such anger."

Eventually, I wore myself out and shut up. I was embarrassed that I was letting this consume me, and talking about it wasn't helping. When I stopped with my outbursts, he started with partial romantics. I woke up to a card on my door. It had a heart on it. I was surprised, but the message pissed me off.

"This may be selfish, but I really miss my friend."

He left one a day at the end of April through the beginning of May. Six said, "I am sorry for the pain I caused." Or something similar. They didn't have the word friend or care; they were touching to me. Every time I saw the word friend or care, it was like a new stab wound.

Honestly, I thought the gesture was so romantic, but the messages were not, so I didn't know what to do or how to feel about this gesture. We do not live close. This meant he dedicated an hour a day to hand-delivering these. The first day they stopped, I was sad. I got used to it. On May 15, he asked if he could bring me something. It was a bag of desserts from my favorite vegan place—three hours away. He said, "I miss you," and handed them to me. I said, "Thank you," and closed the door. I really wanted to let him in. When I opened the bag and saw the strawberry cookie, I thought, OMG, *he is going to make me forget about everything over a cookie.* I fucking love these cookies.

May 25. Issa had a concert; he was there. Issa won an award for going to the all-county chorus, playing in orchestra and regular chorus. I was so proud of him. When it was over, he and Issa were running around and giggling, and I asked myself why. Why is it so tough? When it comes to me and this baby, how come I never feel like we are safe and secure? The sun was setting, and they looked really happy, but none of us were happy. I was lonely, Issa was abandoned by his father, and SWG had his own problems that I didn't understand. But damn, we looked good. Issa had on a crisp dress shirt with a vest, bowtie, and suspenders. SWG had on a black shirt, olive green pants, and the black and olive Retro Nines. I had long lime green and black braids in a bun, a black sweater, black jeans, and crocodile print dress shoes. We all might as well have on tattered rags because of what was happening inside. We just presented well.

I sent out the invites for Issa's graduation in June. SWG called to see if he wanted to see *Spider-Man* as a graduation gift. I respectfully said that he had to go on opening day and he had a play date already, so we settled on *Transformers*. We were not speaking much outside of plans for Issa. Reminded me of what I suppose co-parenting is like. On Issa's big day, he arrived at the house, and everyone waited for Issa to get ready. I had a vision that I wanted him to be surrounded by males because I knew his dad would not be there. His Godfather, both of my brothers, SWG, and myself would be the group. He received a few rewards, and we made a bunch of noise for him. The next stop would be dinner.

While leaving the auditorium, I felt so uncomfortable. I felt a drop of blood on my ankles. Omg. *WHY!* I rushed to the bathroom to fix myself. I was sweating. I returned to the group, and we took pictures outside. My brother said he wasn't coming to dinner because he had to go to work, and before I could roll my eyes, he was gone.

Dinner was at a seafood restaurant on a boating dock patio. The breeze was blowing, and the atmosphere was nice. He offered his arm for me to walk up the stairs because my shoes were so tall. There we are, looking like something again. The server said he paid for dinner, which was cute. Unfortunately, the bleeding was so heavy that I couldn't go straight to the movies and told him I needed to go home. I ran upstairs to wash up and change into jeans. I needed a thick pad; tampons were not holding up. I wouldn't find out until September that I had fibroids causing severe bleeding.

We went to the movies, and Issa's eyes were glued to the screen. He looked at me and put his hand on my tummy. I was going through it. When we got back, I sent Issa to bed. It was a long day, and mommy'ing was over. We sat on the couch, and he was so bold that he put my hand on it. Guess he wasn't shy anymore. He said, "This is how you make me feel." Honestly, I thought that was quite direct and sexy, and if I wasn't bleeding to death, it may have been enough to take me down. He wasn't on my nerves that day, and I liked how we felt.

I said, "I'm not sleeping with you tonight."

That was our pattern; once we started, we could not stop. If he came over, he would stay. He said, "OK." We hugged, and he went home. It might have looked like I had some boundaries; I was just dying and cramping. If he had been my baby for real, I would have loved him to hold me through that agonizing night, but I knew better. I kept my misery to myself and took care of my lady issues by myself.

At the bottom of June, I had mixed emotions; small talk went well, but talking about us was a mess. I was in New York from June 17 to 21. When I was in New York, he left for Europe with his family. He called me while he was at the airport, and I thought that was cute.

On June 23, I had another reading with Miss Rita. She immediately began to speak, and I began to write.

- The smoke was showing a ripple effect, a tornado wind pool of emotion.
- Life or death: speeding things up because I feel as though I'm running out of time.
- Speeding things up can add years to my healing journey.
- She saw the death card. Something has happened, but in your mind, it has not ended.

- This person is a toxic and bad fit for you. Have you asked yourself how can it work; was it me? The ancestors are giving you clear signs; they have given you all the clear signs.
- In your mind, you have created a fairy tale.
- We have been conditioned to believe that we will get the fairy tale ending.
- During the honeymoon phase, it will only take ninety days to reveal what is true.
- This is your year of creation; you will have weeks of creation, and the spirit is working on something just for you.
- You like familiar, and he is familiar, so you keep going through it.
- He is the delay; he is the yellow stop sign.
- Cut him out of your life.
- He is not a good example for your son.
- He is not your husband; you have been hurt several times over. Stop.

Once she was done, I asked some yes and no questions about my mom. Where she wanted her ashes spread, who she wanted them shared with, and if she wanted the house sold or held. Additionally, she had some messages about my siblings. This session had a lot of clarity.

By the time SWG called me again, I was in Turks and Caicos on my first trip without Issa. I went with my sister from another mister, and we had a great time. I had purple down to the booty braids and a full-beat face. When he called, he was in Germany. He told me about his experiences, and I listened. I was smiling a little bit when I got off the phone. By the time he called again, I was at home in bed, and he was in Paris. I would have been really jealous if I hadn't just been there. He showed me the tower in the distance, and I smiled after that call too. I was like, hmm, thinking of me when you're in Paris. . .hmm.

He called at 11:30 p.m. as soon as he got home. He still had his jacket on. He said there were loud alarms at his place, and he couldn't sleep. OK, sir. See you when you get here. I got him some towels so he could decompress in the shower.

He said, "You showering with me?" I said, "I just showered," and he said, "Are you showering with me?"

Now I'm in the shower. I soaped him, we were quiet, and I was wondering if some type of movie scene was going to take place with incredible kissing and passionate wildness. We had been apart from each other for a while, and I was open to some razzle-dazzle. He said he wanted to talk when he got back. So. . .yeah, no. We didn't have sex, and we didn't talk about shit in terms of us. He went to sleep. To top shit off, he seemed annoyed in the morning. He took me to breakfast, but we talked about nothing. It was pretty bad.

July. Things went totally left in July. Issa was out of town. I was kidless, and we could barely coordinate a day or night to be together. Eventually, he invited me to his house for the first time, probably because I had complained that I had never been there. We spoke on the couch for hours before he interrupted me with a kiss. Which I'm never mad at. I couldn't put my finger on it, but something was wrong that night. Although he carried me to the bed, and we kissed each other's private parts, something was wrong. We showered, but it wasn't intimate; we slept, but it wasn't close. When I woke up, he was on the couch and never came back to the room. I said to myself, *Bitch you are crazy; this man does not like you. Do not come back here.*

I called him and said, "Something is wrong," and he said, "Yeah, we should stop." I was annoyed, and I texted later but nothing too crazy. In one of the texts, I told him, "This is lame."

Beautiful Reject, page 12 (Fantasy Theory), was correct; my intuition was correct. Talk to Tash was correct, but I had to fall down a flight of stairs from January to July just to make sure. The lesson here was do not ignore what you already know. If you do not know, stop as soon as you figure it out.

July 17. I started remodeling the guest room. One night, I was tossing and turning in my room, and my cousin, who was staying over in the guest room, came in and said, "Um, the bed in the guest room broke." She was stunned; I was not. I told her she could sleep in my bed. I knew what had to be done. Although we were not communicating, I sensed there was still some negative energy in the house regarding our exchanges not based on love. I was thinking too much about it, and spiritually, there was an internal war about it.

I called a carpenter to repair it. The right leg in the back corner had split. Once it was repaired, I sanded the brown color away and painted the bed black. I repainted the ceiling, and I replaced the ceiling fan. I also went shopping for art with words of encouragement. I painted the curtain rods on the windows black. I added curtain rods to the closet and chose mustard curtains to drape in front of the closet. I found new bedding at Nordstrom that was black and white and inviting. The room looked new and refreshed. The candle that burned the day of the massage dropped on the floor and broke into several pieces. I removed that candle and bought a new one. I open the windows. I burned some sage, and I read some books that belonged to my mother. I was confident that peace would be restored to the space, and it was time to stop making a mountain out of a molehill. That ship had sailed. New space for new experiences.

On July 23, I started a new journey—my prescription from Miss Rita was two weeks of spiritual baths. I found it challenging to sit with myself for long periods of time. By the third day, I missed a bath. My aunt, sister, and I took a trip to Long Island to do a wellness check on my grandpa, and I missed another bath. During my stay, I learned a lot about my family. Originally, my sister was trying to do family portraits, and the main person she wanted to be there was my grandpa. When he couldn't make it, we decided to go to him. I booked double rooms in Long Island and invited my uncles, cousins, and Dad to come.

I heard stories about my mom's childhood. I received pictures of aunts and uncles that I hadn't met. I had a long conversation with my uncle, whom I'd only met once. After this experience, I took a coffee bath. The next day, I had a heated conversation with my grandpa's wife, and I really felt her force. I've seen her several times in the past, but this was the first time I could feel her energy and she could feel mine. It definitely felt like I was in an episode of *Star Wars*.

With things going off track the way they did, by the time I spoke to Rita again on August 6, she gave me some tips and recommended that I start the process over. Tip number one: I'm not supposed to be listening to a bunch of music, doing anything distracting, messing with my hair, or eating popcorn. I'm really just supposed to sit there and think about whatever comes to me or don't think and pray—very simple. I was doing a little bit too much.

August is for Me 2023

I finished making my birthday plans, and I knew that by August, I was going to get the fuck on with it. To have intelligence and not use it is the same as being stupid, and I was being stupid as fuck. I was about to be forty years old! I promised myself three things: I would find things to do all month, I would meet goals throughout the year and consider those achievements as birthday gifts, and I wouldn't link up with anyone on my birthday. Time to move forward. I had a life before these men, and I will have one after. It was time to lay a sturdy foundation that I could build on.

I made a big step. I didn't invite him to anything birthday-related, and I started my no-contact journey. It was time. I had to do better; even with flaws, I deserved better. My man will not play about me; he will be deliberate; he will use words like partner, lover, love, my love, my moon, my center, etc. He will be obvious; he will not be attached to his ex and will be focused on our future; he will be sure (assuming he exists). In the meantime, there are things I could do to make my life comfortable and reduce my anxiety, starting with celebrating my life and healing my mind and my heart.

I moved my celebration with the girls to the weekend of August 14 because I was going to be out of the country on my birthday weekend. Because of this date change, my Aunty Roxy could not come, and I had a fit. I survived and was surrounded by love with a nice brunch in a restaurant with flowers all over the walls. The chef who dropped out of RAE2020 was the owner. He prepared a vegan item for me that was not on the menu; I was all smiles.

That evening, I had dinner at the new AKA hotel with Prince Issa and the friends who couldn't make it to brunch. I booked a suite that I had my eye on. I was not happy that the balcony was not available as that was one of the main reasons I booked the room. It had a green wet bar and a living room, and I spent the night with Prince Issa! I felt really good when I went to bed. My friends got me some very thoughtful gifts. I felt loved. Now that my local tradition had taken place, it was time to get ready for Africa.

The motivation for this trip was rooted in an invitation to a wedding. I met the bride at Shenandoah University in 2016 while working in the business office. We welcomed her on a full scholarship for her Master's in Business. She spoke four languages and displayed pristine problem-solving skills in statistics and accounting.

During our preparations for the annual business symposium, she said, "If I get married, would you come?" I said, "Of course." After departing SU, we kept in touch through Hair Therapy services. I started her locs and styled her daughter's hair.

COVID affected everything. She got married, yet assured me I did not miss the party and the notable shindig would be in Tanzania at their traditional ceremony. I received the invite well in advance. I am ashamed to say I didn't start putting things in motion for the trip until the month before. My dad's dream was to visit the Serengeti, and I made sure to include him in my plans.

Issa wants to be a pilot; he makes model planes and always shares his knowledge of aircraft with me. I was searching for our flights based on the aircraft of his dreams. A flight on the A380 with Emirates. I looked forward to seeing the look on his face. He said, "Mom, really?" He started recording immediately, but then had the nerve to ask why he didn't have an engine view, aka business class seat. I reminded myself he thinks in experiences and not dollars and told him to get happy and grateful fast. It was a long fifteen-hour flight.

The compound in Dar, where the bride and groom stayed, would be my home away from home for the duration of the trip. It was designed as a vacation home. We stayed in a wing that had three suites. Each room had a full bathroom and AC. I had an affinity for the hallway designed with lush curtains and a wall-sized mirror.

The front yard was huge, with a pool, lush garden, basketball court, and two tables. The main house held the kitchen, living room, and additional bedrooms. There was security and a groundskeeper at all times. A cook was present for most of our stay.

Our itinerary was packed, and after a long day of international flights, we woke up the next morning for a domestic flight to Kilimanjaro. Once we arrived, a driver took us to AIM Mall. We met the co-owner of our touring company, and he introduced us to Eric, our tour guide for the next few days. Eric took us straight to Tarangire Park.

Safari Day One

I bought things almost everywhere. My guide did not recommend the gift shop at Tarangire Park. After a few experiences, I learned the value of not getting too excited and buying the first thing I saw. Many of the same items are available within the region at better prices. Buying too many overpriced trinkets would deplete the souvenir budget. We stopped at a roadside Maasai shop; it was a tad pricey, and they expected me to haggle. I bought two bracelets for $8 each. It was fascinating to see the woodworking and painting being done behind the shop.

Jambo Tanzania is a new development that took my breath away. It was the most shoppable complex ever. The prices were reasonable. I would later find similar earrings and bracelets at a lower cost, but that shopping experience included being heckled while walking in the streets. I was slightly unsure of my safety and sense of direction. At Jambo, the sales reps spoke both Swahili and English. The layout was open and spacious. The new complex houses the newest location of the House of Gems. I was able to touch the precious stone tanzanite I had been dreaming of for the first time here. I danced joyfully with Eric as my dad signed the paperwork for the triangle earrings he bought me.

Safari Day Two

Maasai Village, aka shake-down town. This is a well-thought-out tourist shake-down spot. If you choose to stop at a village, you must spend $50 USD to enter. The chief will tell you this about five minutes after saying hello while walking to the entrance. After you agree and pay the fee, they wrap a cloth on you and perform a welcome song.

Once you enter the village, you are taken to tour a hut. When you leave the hut, you are escorted to a table of souvenirs, starting with souvenirs made by the owners of the house you were in. Once you collect the things you like, a village woman gives the total. The quote was $166! For a plate, a bowl, and a bracelet. I asked for only the bracelet, and that was $20!—the most expensive bead bracelet from my entire trip. The same or similar bracelet is $7 in shops and $2 on the street.

Then they ask if you want to see the school. There is a huge donation box there. The children say some words and math operations in Swahili. The chief asks, "Would you like to donate money to the school?" If you put money in the box, the children clap. Then you walk back to the car, where they remove the cloth from you. We were there for about 30 minutes and spent $90.

We visited The Arusha Cultural Heritage Centre, which is enormous, and no pictures are allowed inside the art gallery section. The art is creative; one piece took forty years to make. This is the largest art gallery in East Africa. The Heritage Centre has a huge multi-level gift shop.

On the second floor, there is a jewelry shop where you will find the owner showcasing alluring rings, earrings, and bracelets. They accept Visa for purchases of tanzanite. Discover is not accepted in Tanzania. US cash, shillings, and Visa are the most common forms of payment. The certificate for tanzanite includes information on the cut, weight, and clarity. More information is included on the Heritage Centre certificate of authenticity than the House of Gems. Paperwork is required to take tanzanite back to the US. If questioned and you do not have paperwork, it may be confiscated. I didn't want that to happen to me.

Zanzibar

To get to Zanzibar, we took the ferry, which was a wild experience. When the car pulled up, men touched the car like Beyonce was inside. They tell you they are an official worker and to follow them. They harass you to carry your bag and demand a specific tip of $15 each. I did not buy my ticket in advance. My dad opted for gold, the step above economy, for $50 each. We liked not being out in the elements with AC. The ride was smooth and peaceful. The hounding for taxis and hustling to purchase products resumed as soon as we arrived in Stone Town.

The lesson I learned in Zanzibar is that no guide equals no fun. On day one, we walked from the hotel to the Freddie Mercury Museum. The museum was informative but small for the price; it took about fifteen minutes to complete. We tried to sit in Forodhani Park on the way back, but that was not relaxing. We were constantly approached by people selling things from boat rides to photos. A man even told Issa it was $5 to play on a public beat-up playground that was clearly free.

We called Cholo, a guide the bride recommended. He met us at the hotel, and we walked back to the same park, but it felt different. He spoke to everyone but no one spoke to us.

It was great! I decided to get my henna done because it was something I wanted to have for the wedding. I paid $25, and the locals told me that was way too much. We experienced the infamous Forodhani street food market that takes place every night. Cholo was in charge of our experience for day two. He took us to the following places.

1. Nungwi Natural Aquarium
2. Nungwi Beach
3. Kwale Island
4. Sandbar near Kwale Island
5. Mangrove near Kwale Island

The aquarium was small, informative, and fun. Nungwi Beach looked amazing, but the shores felt rocky. Local men rent the chairs, and the Maasai walk the beach fully robed, asking, "Are you OK?" I assume people often ask to take pictures with them, and then they charge them. The ride to get on the boat to Kwale was an hour. Walking to the boat over the low tide was an experience. The boat ride was pleasant, and plenty of fruits were served. The diver diving to get starfish was a highlight for me.

Kwale Beach was active. I ate fruit from a 300-year-old Baobab tree. We picked up food from Kwale, and the sandbar was a short ride away. Cholo's crew pitched a tent for shade. The food was excellent. My dad said it was a bad-ass meal; that means it was really good. The mangrove waters are still, quiet, low, and warm. For the finale, they raised the sails of the Dhow boat. The wind carried us back quicker than the motor. As the boat sailed over the seas, I told myself, "I am on the Indian Ocean with my dad and my little Prince. I am so happy I made this happen." In the midst of my joy, I felt fear. I was in a tiny boat; what happens if I fall out? OMG, get me back to shore. To distract myself, I took a selfie, holding up my big bun made with forest green braids.

Saturday, August 26, was the main event, my friend's wedding. We were late to the church. Even though we were late, there were still three additional hours before the "I do." Five sets of brides got married at the same time. I wasn't familiar with that custom, but they watched each other take vows and walked out of the church together. There was a fancy car with flowers for each bride, and they were welcomed by the community and guests. The reception was white and gold and grand, with over thirty tables and a white dance floor. Different tribes were called to the front to do their dance. Money was presented to the bride and the groom. Everyone in the family gave speeches. And the MC kept the party going. We danced to Master KG "Jerusalema Feat. Nomcebo," and every time I hear that song, I think of that amazing night. I practiced for a few weeks to make sure I didn't mess up the dance.

They invited people who had traveled from far to the front to present them with cakes. It was my first traditional African wedding, and I loved it. I was proud of my friend for showing her strength and endurance. Some customs and traditions took place days before I arrived and continued days after I left. She smiled through everything and said that she was so happy. She looked like an angel. Her locs were in an updo with pearls. Her makeup was perfect, and her off-the-shoulder dress was custom-made. We stayed up late that night recapping events from the day. When I rose the next day, I felt bittersweet about my African adventure ending.

Heading back while sitting on the plane, I realized the layover was four hours, unlike the one-and-a-half hours coming. Just enough time to squeeze in the Burj Khalifa if we left the airport right way. I read that the building was fifteen minutes from the airport.

Dubai's Airport was huge. It was a lot of walking. Also, the staff was forceful about shuffling people to the connecting flight area. When I asked how to leave the airport, one staff member told me I could not. I knew that was not true. I asked another staff member for directions to the exit. He told me to make sure I was back an hour before and told me where to go. We arrived at 9:30 p.m. and were outside with our carry-ons by 10:30 p.m.

Once we were picked up by the taxi, we hit the highway and marveled at the signs in another language. Our taxi driver was kind, giving us information about everything we saw. When we arrived at the Burj Khalifa, Issa gasped, jumped out of the car, and started taking pictures. He said something along the lines of, "It's a beauty."

I love his enthusiasm for architecture, and I knew that if it wasn't for him, I wouldn't be there. At that moment, I felt blessed to be chosen as his mother and guide in this life. Although sometimes I feel he is my guide and I'm just the chaperone because he's underage. He has led me to explore places that were not top of mind and reminded me that the only barrier is thinking I can't do something.

We returned just before midnight for our flight that departed at 2 a.m. Security made me reprint my boarding pass because it had ripped in my purse. Issa lost track of his bag at the Emirates passport checkpoint. I had to go back to get it; those fifteen minutes of not having the carry-on with all the essentials were stressful.

Once we boarded, it was a smooth flight home, and we marveled at the excitement of adding Dubai to an already great trip. I dreamed about the sexy Chanel suit I saw in the airport for most of the flight home. Time was going backward as it was my birthday again on the plane. They brought me chocolates with rose petals and three glasses of nectar for us to toast. They also took a picture of the three of us with a Polaroid. How nostalgic.

It was August 28 in America, and I had little to no energy. There was a bit of a mishap in securing the cake I wanted, and I ended up with nothing. I went across the street and bought a vegan cupcake from a new bakery that opened. It looked good for the picture when the family sang to me, but it tasted horrible. My auntie brought me a dozen red roses, and my son presented me with a live portrait he drew, and it looked so good. He captured my big bun and earrings. His gifts always touch my core. I was smiling big. Finally, a trip where I wasn't thinking about men and what should have been and dissecting washed-up scenarios. I was present; I enjoyed my son, my dad, and my family, and I was ready to take charge and be a boss-ass bitch. No more wounded bird. I was ready to maintain no contact and clear my mind.

Issa already missed the first week of school; we had one night of rest and had to get with the program. He wanted to try a sport this year and was displeased to learn he had missed soccer tryouts. I even did my usual complaining, and they still wouldn't let him try out for the team.

CHAPTER 7

SEPTEMBER 2023 - 2024
THE YEAR OF THE ROSE

    This year, my Aunt Sharon visited and shared in the remembrance of my mom. September 2 was a refulgent day. We went to get manicures and to the MGM Casino at the National Harbor to see their garden art installation. We took tons of pictures, and it was nice to be smiling. We had burgers and people watched. Aunty was down for a road trip, and on September 4, she, Issa, and I revisited Ginter Botanical Garden. It was jazz day and we enjoyed live music for hours.

    After the garden, we enjoyed The Hop Craft Pizza. While Aunty was visiting, I made things I don't usually make, such as salmon or other seafood. Aunty also likes music; her nineties hits were bumping out of her pink JBL speaker all the time. After Aunty left, I found a new project to embark on.

    I started construction on the closet in my bedroom. I removed the popcorn ceiling, changed the color from beige to white, then shopped for stainless steel rods. The first rod went up with no problem. The second rod gave me a hard time. I thought the rod was secure, but when I let go, it fell to the ground and sliced the side of my leg. I was angry. I wanted to do something for myself and didn't foresee an injury so early in the project. I took the night, regrouped, and tried again in the morning.

I had to modify the design because one of the old brackets I had removed wasn't compatible with the new rod. After some tweaking, I was finally done, and my closet looked crisp, clean, and refreshed like the rest of my room. My finishing touch was a Wi-Fi-enabled light bulb that could change color. These projects really held my focus and used my mind for critical thinking that wasn't attached to emotions or romantic complications. The smallest project still has a way of turning the whole house upside down. Taking breaks from overanalyzing my life was restorative.

It was Self-Care September and time to revisit the baths that I had a hard time with. The assignment was seven days of dark baths, aka coffee baths. I set up an altar for my mom in the hallway with her and my grandma's photos, a few candles, and a cup of water. It was day one, and although I wasn't looking forward to the bath, I was looking forward to the outcome, so I sat there. I didn't do anything; I listened to the water and whatever thoughts came through my head until the timer for thirty minutes went off. I got up, and I was so proud of myself at this first bath.

Dark Spiritual Baths Round 2

Day One. I thought about East Fortieth Street, where I used to live, the physical abuse that I saw as a child, and the times I got in trouble as a child. I thought of my paternal grandpa standing by his bookcase and many other things.

Day Two. More thoughts about my childhood in Brooklyn around the fifth grade.

Day Three. The day I was injured trying to fix my closet. I had a huge bruise on my leg; I was pretty upset. I thought the bath would calm me down, but I was still frustrated. I thought about my own sexual abuse. I was sad, and that was uncomfortable. Sad about sex in general. I thought about The Home Depot.

Day Four. I thought about a hymn I used to sing in church called *Greet Somebody in Jesus' Name* when I was nine and lived in Tobago. I thought about the time a roommate stole my underwear in college. I thought about sex; I thought about the sexual assault again. My stepmom, whom I missed significantly, and why she didn't reach out after I shared that my mom passed. I thought about when I said goodbye to her for the last time when I returned to America. Thought about my mom's diary I had found. I was so excited and thought I would learn more about her, only to find out she wrote only on the first few pages. Then I got a little nervous after I heard some sounds.

Day Five. Thought about my cousin who lived in New York. And I thought of the song, "Love Lifted Me," another song that I used to sing in the choir in church when I was a child.

Day Six. The hymn, "Love Lifted Me." I heard the name Agatha. I heard the phrase *daughter of gold*. I took deep breaths, and my shoulders felt heavy. I heard the name again. Agatha Hopkinson. That's it.

Day Seven. During my bath, I sang the entire time, mostly hymns "Kumbaya," "Love Lifted Me," "Let Your Living Water Flow," "Lift Every Voice," "Amazing Grace," and finally, "Let the Flowers Bloom Again" by Denyse Plummer. I also read Psalm 91. There was a rocking motion in the water.

Rita did a reading at the end of the seven days that confirmed I was on the right path. There was a mother card showing support, and it was time to work on my crown chakra and break cycles. Take calming baths for clarity on issues that came up in dark baths. They are soothing. I was sick of soaking. I was excited at the thought of a white bath because the dark baths could get very intense. They were unpredictable. Sometimes, they gave you a few thoughts, and sometimes, it seemed like it presented every thought you ever had. I was ready to compare the experiences.

White Spiritual Baths

Day One. Iceland and how wondrous it was. Thought about floating in the water in the Lagoon. I paid attention to the water in the tub and how I couldn't see through it. Constantly moving my hand up and down from visibility to invisible.

Day Two. My mom's last words, "Candice." That was the only thought I had—my name.

Day Three. I had chest pain, stretched my legs. I stretched and stretched. I thought of One with Ebony.

Day Four. More stretching. Made tornadoes in the water, watched it twirl, and focused on it.

Day Five. I closed my eyes and leaned back. I rocked back and forth, back and forth; my hands were open palm up (receiving hands). The messages are received, be still in the midst of chaos, try not to talk for the rest of the night.

Day Six. My shoulders felt scaly. I received, "You will shed layers so you can run." Hummed and focused on my knees.

Every time I was assigned these baths, I would end up in New York. Day seven fell on September 23, Grandma's birthday. The house is forty years old and the bathroom was icky. I got some gloves and scrubbed. I made sure everything was as clean as it could be before I started this bath. I found a picture of my grandpa and lit white candles.

Additionally, my therapist gave me an assignment to write a letter to my father, a response to a letter that he wrote to me in college when he was in rehab for alcoholism. I pulled the note to the side and told myself that after my bath, I'd share this with my dad.

Day Seven. The water is hot and not calming. I saw glowing white lights. I sat there and thought, *This is it*. This has to be the equivalent of the first time a student breaks a board in karate class. I watched the little white lights until they disappeared and took a deep breath. Then I prepared to read the letter to my dad.

"Hey, Dad, you wrote me this letter when I was in college, and my therapist thought it would be very healing for you if I responded to it now that I am an adult. She questioned why I always sing your praises and whether there was anything that's ever happened that bothered me. Initially, I said, 'No, I love my daddy.' She challenged me to think longer. I recollect the time when I didn't have access to you for six months without explanation—that was scary. After six months, you sent your letter, I felt relief."

I read to my daddy line by line a response to everything that he told me. I assured him that no mistake he could ever make could reduce my amount of love for him. No relationship with the woman (even if I love her) is more important to me than my relationship with him. He was misty-eyed, and he asked me to make sure to leave my letter on his desk, which made me smile.

Another reason I love therapy is because it makes you think about where troubles started and how to end them. I don't believe this is something I've been carrying with me, but she believed it's something that he may be carrying. It was important for me to remember that parents carry burdens too. Just like I do for Issa, my parents have some for me.

When I shared my experience with Rita, she told me that the water feeling hot is symbolic of shedding and that it's unusual for white baths to be hot. I finally did it. I put a check next to having some discipline, intention, focus, and the ability to self-heal. I was sure that was Grandpa. I had seen many images of him in my dreams and the baths.

Miss Ellen

I felt great sorrow when I learned of the passing of one of my former clients. I met her through her niece in 2013. We didn't speak often, and one day, she sent a word of encouragement when I was thinking about discontinuing writing the Hair Therapy Newsletter.

How wonderful a person must be to be sick and still make time to check on others. In subsequent messages, she shared that she was proud of the mom I've become and happy that I traveled to Iceland with Issa. I always kept her in mind going forward and told myself that if my one reader was Miss Ellen, that would be enough for me. I wrote about her and shared her photos. She was an amazing woman.

"It is with great sadness that I announce Hair Therapy has gained an angel. Miss Ellen Conley-Green III transitioned on September 19, 2023. She was a respected veteran and a leader, loved by her family, community, and coworkers. I am grateful to have known her. In her honor, I will write about restaurants and healthy food in the November Newsletter."

I attended her funeral with a hole in my chest. I wanted to speak, but I was too shy. She told me she had cancer. I told her I would visit, and I did not. I had more than enough time to take Issa to see her. I regretted not making a bigger effort to be there for her. I wept quietly when I saw the announcement. The tears of guilt fell before the tears of sorrow.

When everyone left the funeral, I walked to her casket. "Miss Ellen, forgive me. I am so sorry; Issa and I are here now. You will be missed."

Grandma's Birthday 2023

My grandma was turning ninety-one this year. I arrived on her birthday at 10 a.m. The first item on the list was to buy her a beautiful dress. I sent my dad some pictures, and he picked an emerald lace dress. It came with a jacket and a brooch, and she reminded me of Queen Elizabeth. We had a few more people attend than the year before, and the house was full of joy and music. This year, Issa's bow tie was green to match his grandma's dress, and my hair was green and black as well. We were taking the match with Grandma thing very far. Grandma really couldn't stay awake this year, and it was hard to get a photo of her smiling.

We ended September attending my friend's fortieth birthday party. We were dressed to the nines, and Issa was the only kid in the building. I really had to have a talk with myself. *Girl, you cannot take your child everywhere.* He brought her a really great gift, and we left early to let the grown-ups have their time.

October started with two birthday celebrations for my friend's moms, and Issa delivered roses for both occasions—fuchsia frosted roses for the first and burnt orange roses for the second. This month, I wasn't as exhausted from self-care and was ready to take the next steps. I took my first in-person spiritual bath with Miss Rita.

Before the bath, I was required to sit in a room by myself and collect my thoughts. It is acquired after the bath to wear white. As a person who's been wearing black since 2015, I had to shop for this outfit. When she took my photo, I paused because I saw my momma's face again. When I came home, I rushed to the visitor's room to take a picture beside my mommy. I didn't feel sorrow; this was the closest I had felt to her since she passed.

Issa was having trouble with his music; he was starting to forget the notes. He wasn't practicing as much. I reached out to his instructor to see if he would do an in-home session, and he said he was open to it. Dr. G spent hours giving Issa a great refresher course. My favorite part of the lesson was when he showed Issa examples of different musical styles, and I got to listen to how talented Dr. G is.

October always seemed to be the month that I literally let my hair down. This was a time when I remembered what I looked like without braids that go down to my waist. One of the reasons I don't wear my hair out often is because when I have my natural hair, I look so much like my mom. I'm not sure how one can have imposter syndrome with looking like their mom, but I have it. When my hair is colored and outrageous, it shows more of my personality and not stealing Momma's look. There is no way for me to look in the mirror and not think of her when I see my natural gray and black hair, and sometimes it's overwhelming.

In November, I was in for a surprise when Dad told me that he was going to London. I go places all the time, but now I was on the receiving end of him going someplace without me. I was happy for him to be having fun, but I missed him so much knowing he wasn't in New York, just four hours away. He always told me the story of my first birthday in London; I had two birthdays, one in London and one in America. I have a great aunt and cousin there, but I haven't been since.

November 11 was the day that I took a goat milk and rose petal bath. This was specifically to calm my nerves and ease my mind. My altar received some upgrades. I had an amethyst rock and my Mickey Mouse cup with coffee. My rock fell, and four pieces broke off. At first, I was vexed, but then I interpreted it symbolically. I decided I would start using each rock to represent a member of my family: myself, my brother, my sister, and my son, and the rock bed itself representing my mother and my ancestors.

On this day, after completing my recommended bath, I needed to get ready to record the interviews for RAE2024. My brother was outside of the house unannounced. He texted that he would need to move in earlier that morning, and I had no response. This brought great stress upon me. To avoid panic, I left the house out the back door so that I could go to the studio in peace without increasing my heart rate by trying to have a conversation with him about it. A few days later, I started looking for houses. The family home on paper was too complex. Still in Mom's name and deeded to three people. I lived there and paid the bills, but I was always on the brink of a sibling mentioning moving "home."

The Year of Responsibility

I intended to get a home very close to the family home, and I quickly realized that new construction in my area was not affordable for my salary. I pivoted from looking at the nearby expensive condos to townhomes further south, about forty minutes. On November 18, I went to look at a community recommended by a loan officer and fell in love with the model, the Strauss. That was the street my grandma's house was on in Brooklyn. Based on my salary, the sales rep said I could be preapproved. I called my real estate agent friend, and she went back with me on November 21.

The loan officer said upon further review that I could not get the Strauss but that I qualified for the Clarendon. She told me I could start the process by putting $1,000 down. I had to walk through the model one more time because the Strauss was really what I was going for. I told myself it's my first home, not my forever home; it's all about affordability. I gave her the $1,000, and she gave me the sold sticker. The sold sticker was a bit aggressive because many different steps needed to be cleared to make that "sold" a reality. Nonetheless, Issa and I took the picture smiling in front of lot H with the sold sticker.

As the weeks passed, I was inspired to expand my altar with more candles. I also took time to write in a journal and leave it there. I declared the upcoming year to be the year of responsibility. We were leaving the year of travel. The first sacrifice I needed to make to secure closing was to reduce my spending and decrease my credit card balances. They gave me a folder with my floor plan, and I used the white space at the bottom of the floor plan to make my new monthly budget. I broke my budget into percentages as my good friend Dr.Rufaro, who saved my momma's house, advised. Fifty, thirty, and twenty.

- 50 percent for needs
- 30 percent for wants
- 20 percent for savings

That was the structure I had been using for the past year. The modification: wants were reduced to 10 percent—just enough to keep getting my hair done, and I used the 20 percent toward my earnest deposit. I paid $1,000 a month toward my earnest deposit until May. A perk of new construction. To think I was going to start looking for a place in April. If all went well, I would be closing in July or August. I put it in my mind that the house was a birthday gift to myself and my son. For his birthday, we would not be traveling around the world, and for my birthday, I would celebrate a spa concept that I dreamed of in my new house.

December was about studying, cooking, eating at home as much as possible, and making outings minimal. Issa was on the principal's honor roll, and maintaining those grades was no easy feat. It required at least two hours of after-school work every day to keep up with the assignments and teaching him in areas where he needed assistance. Eating out was the death of the budget and our favorite pastime. It was quite an adjustment.

Issa had a beautiful winter concert led by a Black teacher who looked just like him. They sang a song called "Hot Chocolate," and I was mesmerized. She had every grade level up there jamming, singing their part, and doing their hand dances. It reminded me of many moons ago when I was in choir, and it was enjoyable. I did not invite SWG and I was OK with that. I also disconnected from him on social media, which was helpful. I realized how much leaving the door open in that manner wasn't as nurturing for us as I thought it would be. It was keeping Issa and me hopeful for more. After the concert, Issa told me "Hot Chocolate" was the most exhilarating performance of his life. He appeared exuberant.

I took pride in adding flowers to my altar. I also had an ironing board with an African cloth that I used as an additional altar with my mom's ashes and photos of her. The hallway was a space where Issa and I would talk openly about our feelings and how much we missed her. The space to acknowledge her allowed us to address our pain of her not being there in the physical form.

We ended the year with a bang at Auntie Roxy's New Year's Eve party. I didn't know I could have so much fun inside the house. The tables were dressed in silver, black, and gold. The food table was festive and tiered. I loved that her events looked professional and that she put all that energy into the family.

Academic Advocacy for Prince Issa

In January, it seemed I was at Issa's school every day, but it was more like once a week. Inquiring about how assignments were graded or why assignments were missing. They would say, "It's the child's responsibility to complete the assignments. Allow Issa to be independent." And I would respond, "It's my responsibility to make sure that he is OK." Nothing they would tell me would ever make me back down. I've had grading systems changed as I questioned the weighting of assignments and the structure of assignments for children. I called attention to notification systems. Identified teachers who didn't provide material to make it easy for parents to follow along. I challenged any negative comments on report cards that weren't addressed with the parent before the end of the marking period. I was a force to be reckoned with.

Sometimes, they would bring up his age as though that was a factor. Programs are competitive when they look at you on paper—they're looking for extensive writing skills, the highest GPA, and who referred you to the program. I knew who the competition would be, and I wanted to make sure Issa had the best advantage for his interest in aviation. Aviation requires a solid mathematical foundation. Issa disproportionately spends time mastering it.

At ten years old, I became lost in the subject of math. I could never catch up because I didn't have anyone making sure I understood the material beyond in-class instruction. I purchased the software they use at school; it's intuitive and checks for incorrect answers. At home, Issa completed the assigned work a second time to retain information or if he worked ahead of the class.

I used Khan Academy on YouTube and hired private tutors to make sure Issa kept up. I turned my ears off to the staff and their advice because it sounded like they were telling us to strive to be mediocre, and that was not an option for us. His dreams require rigorous preparation, and his at-home education team understood that.

January 5, 2023. I was at a party bragging about my son, which led to a recommendation for a potential mentor for Issa. He was invited to the Wings of Legacy Celebration, pioneering stories of Black aviation past and present. He met with Herbert Jones III, the son of former Tuskegee airman Herbert H. Jones, Jr. I stood back and smiled as my son held his own in a very mature conversation about aeronautic events in history. This was one of the first times that it hit me. My son is not in a phase. Little boys have phases: cars, trains, planes, and dinosaurs. It seemed he was where he belonged on the path to his calling.

January 15. Issa was invited to the advanced chorus by his chorus teacher. He went on to perform at a Delta coordinated event, the Martin Luther King Oracle competition. He was awarded a certificate of service. Issa's enthusiasm for music placed him on his chorus teacher's husband's radar. Issa gained a pending invite to join the Kappa League the subsequent year. By the end of January, we received startling news that the choir teacher would be leaving at the end of the year.

I spent the bottom half of January on the internet promoting RAE2024. I was informed that my mentor could make it, and he would be this year's guest speaker. It was very important to me that this event was worthy in the material and aesthetics of his trip from Africa and sponsorship. I hadn't been this nervous in a long time.

January 22, 2023. I encouraged Issa to journal with me on my mom's birthday. I knew that he missed her so much that sometimes it was hard to talk about it.

RAE2024

February, I did not sleep much. I spent my days visiting the RAE2024 participants at their places of work to get B-roll footage of their daily lives. I spent my nights putting the documentary together and going over every detail and transition of the event. The event was on February 24, and I worked every day to ensure it went well.

I visited the Social Justice School in DC to highlight the principal for the documentary. I visited WETA, and to support the previous year's participants, we went to the presentation, "His Story of the Drum" by Jason, in which Malik DOPE participated. The information in it was informative and riveting. The presentation was comprised of poetry, various drums, and African dance performances. Producers asked Issa for his on-camera feedback after the show.

I became a part of a book club that I was invited to after meeting another enthusiastic mom with a vegan shirt on at a PTA meeting. I was enjoying my time with this new circle of women dedicated to furthering education for their children.

I posted about RAE day and night. Just one week shy of the event, Issa had breakouts on his back and a scar on his lip. Another obstacle was that the Angelika Theater system could not read movie files. The movie had to be in DCP format, which I was unfamiliar with. I watched YouTube University for forty-eight hours to learn how to do this conversion. I considered having someone else do it, but the turnaround time was too long, and the cost was completely out of my budget. I was up until 3 a.m. the night before waiting for the file to render and hoping the conversion worked. I could not confirm if it was playable at home because my computer can't read DCP files. I had to wait until the morning of the event.

My makeup, dress, and hair were flawless. I stayed at a nearby hotel to reduce any problems of getting stuck in traffic. I was running a little late, so I parked in front. Thirty minutes out, we had a few items that needed to be taken from the hotel to the theater. My aunt called and told me my car would not start. I stepped out of the hotel, confirmed the car would not start, and started walking in the rain to my event. My heart was pounding out of my chest. I forgot several things: my jewelry (the earrings dad bought me) and the net still on my bun. I received many compliments, and the people supporting me, such as my Aunt Roxy and the chef Shayla, put out many fires that were not public facing. Everything looked perfect. Behind the scenes, it was a complete shit show.

The volunteers in charge of BTS were having a tough time. One of the volunteers walked around with the camera but did not take any photos. It was upsetting to discover that after the event was almost over. No one took video footage of my mentor saying that he loved me and was proud of me, and I was so upset. My phone was dying. Video coverage wasn't going well overall.

On-screen, the documentary was captivating. I was proud of myself. The only thing that really ground my gears was in the credits, where I noticed I had spelled the word photographer wrong. I wanted to jump into a hole. I wanted it to be flawless. Overall, it was great. People came dressed up. Everybody had their suits and gowns and looked amazing. Black educators, a

Nike rep, and so many different organizations and entrepreneurs were represented that night. My crowd was around the same number of people, forty to fifty, but I could see that the crowd matured and was diverse.

I was grateful for the previous participants who sent their clips in to update viewers on what they had been working on. Prince Issa made his appearance and had his usual reaction. This time, he was bold and spoke into the camera. I love that he said, "If my mom chose you, that means you are doing good."

When it was almost over, I was trembling. SWG was there. He sent a significant donation. I didn't expect to be so nervous when I saw him. We did not speak much, only for one minute from the theater door to the red carpet. I wasn't sure if I was having a panic attack or a spiritual awakening at the end of the event, and seeing him didn't help. I darted out after the closing announcements at the same time he did. He was also walking very fast. Usually, I would have coordinated taking group photos or mingling. I still can't believe that happened. Afterward, my aunt said people were wondering where I went. I was standing on the red carpet, catching my breath from the foot race. They eventually found me.

My mentor told me a long time ago that sometimes, when we shake and tremor, nothing is wrong with us. It is us moving to the next level. I think I may have moved to the next level that day. Just days before the event, my mentor's business partner died in a plane crash. He revealed in his speech that he was supposed to be on that plane, and I gasped. I could not imagine my life without him in it. These gatherings were becoming more than highlighting the life of the living. I could see that it may not be the last time that we told the story of someone we'd tragically and unexpectedly lost.

Recovering from RAE took about a week. I was very tired. The lesson: hire the photographer. We had a little bit of surplus, and if I had spent it on a photographer or videographer, I might have prevented the heart attack I was having trying to be cute and polite while I wanted to say, *Someone fucking record these moments because they are not going to happen again.*

Hello!!!

The Exorcism

In March, Issa started getting scars and bumps on his body. I took him to the dermatologist, and she prescribed some medication. The scars and the breakouts did not stop, and I called Miss Rita. I told her that I was concerned for Issa. His skin is paper smooth, and I've never seen anything like this before. She suggested a spiritual bath for him. I was nervous about letting him do it by himself, so I opted to do one also. It would be my second time and his first. She left us in the room with the blue light to talk about anything on our minds.

Issa expressed to me that he wanted a family, and he wanted his parents to be together. My eyes were enlarged. I said, "I can't be with your dad, baby." He said he wanted me to be with someone new who doesn't give up on us. I asked him if he was talking about SWG, and he said yes. He was really harboring feelings and worry over my tension with his dad and me finding love.

Earlier in the year (December), Issa and his dad were texting, and he invited him to my house without telling me. His dad showed up on my doorstep unannounced after being missing since Issa's tenth birthday. I scolded Issa and felt a bit betrayed. After that, I set up a session for his dad to meet with Issa's therapist. She could assess if he was sound and plan how to reintroduce him into Issa's life. I attended the session, and we made a plan. Issa was to write his feelings for the therapist and then have a session with his dad to express his feelings when I wasn't present. His dad came to the intake with me and did not show up at the session where Issa was supposed to share his feelings. He said he forgot and had to work. Issa was crestfallen. I blocked him. Issa's therapist called him several times, and he never called her back.

Issa's desire to have a dad of his own or a father-figure, plus blaming himself for the tension, was manifesting in him physically, making him sick. He took his bath with herbs and the African drums playing in the background and markings on his face, definitely looking like a participant in the Busta Rhymes nineties, "Put Your Hands Where My Eyes Can See."

The next unexpected thing happened when Rita noticed that her snake had an interest in Issa. She asked if Issa would like to hold it, and he said yes. I know Issa to be afraid of most things, including dogs, and I was very surprised. My son held the snake with a smile on his face. He was so calm and said, "Mom, I feel lighter." He went home and slept for six hours.

Another major concern was that Issa was twirling his hair and pulling pieces of it out. I had been struggling with this quietly for some time, camouflaging the broken pieces, twisting and reattaching his locs. But it seemed it was getting out of control, and I needed help. I hoped that this bath would help with that.

Later that week, Issa hosted his first art event with all the little kids in our life. We painted different shapes of pottery, ice cream cones, animals, and jeeps and then baked them. The kids enjoyed that. The woman at the establishment kept asking whose birthday it was. She couldn't wrap her head around the fact that we were hosting a community event that didn't revolve around being born.

I continue to enhance and grow my altar, adding four to five candles and consistently changing the floral arrangements. I also attended therapy in person for the first time in a long time. My insurance required me to go once a year. My therapist told me how proud she was of my progress and how much I had grown since the first time she saw me. She drew a diagram on her whiteboard that read, "Your body knows the score."

At the top was the word "acceptance," and she drilled into me how important it was to accept exactly what a person was saying. Do not jump to conclusions. Having too much cortisol in my body would make me sick. At the end of the session, we took a picture in front of the angel wings. The angel wings were a donation from one of her international modeling friends. She gave me a little sticker that looked like a light bulb and told me to write something important. I wrote, "No serial dating." I had not been, but it was a good reminder.

March 20. My son and I showed up to track tryouts late. I'm running on the field with a computer in my hand because I'm technically working the late shift at work. I looked absolutely ridiculous, but I was trying really hard to make sure he didn't miss this opportunity. He raced against a kid who smoked him pretty bad. I wondered if that was an indication of whether he would be accepted. The coach allowed him to be on the team. She was checking to see if Issa would give up, which he did not. The test was not about how fast he could run but whether he believed in himself. A few other kids who had been trying out for two days were cut and did not receive the pink welcome paper.

March 25. Dr. Davis invited me to the University of Southern California, where they hosted "Africa Engages the

Diaspora." I sat quietly at the table, listening to various global presentations about the state of African Americans and the diaspora. It was enlightening. I used to try to keep my worlds separate, my entrepreneurship life from my educational career. I thought everything had to be divided.

This year taught me that, from looking at the audience at RAE to the invites that I had received lately, I can be many things at once. I can be a fashionista with eclectic earrings who's educated and confident in what she's speaking about, whether it's movies, my natural opinion on any given topic, or my son's education. I did not have to disguise myself. There is no need to hide myself. I can show indicators of my personality in every realm. I sat at this table with the biggest Afro in the room, and I felt free. No braids. No bob. I felt this meeting called for an Afro. The thought that people would say the way we were born isn't professional is so upsetting sometimes. But I digress. I wore my Shenandoah pin proudly on my lapel.

By the end of this month, one of the locs in the front of Issa's hair fell out; I was mortified. I reevaluated our diet. I ordered vitamins and showered him with love.

April had an unexpected revelation in it. I went to the former Hair Therapy location to catch up with the current owner, who is also my former stylist. I hadn't seen her in a while, and I wanted my hair done for Issa's birthday. I wanted that touch that you can only get from her.

We spoke, and she asked me how I had been doing. She mentioned that she had heard some unsettling things during the transition and the end of the Hair Therapy era. She spoke to me about my behavior and some things I said. I couldn't recall much of it, but she didn't miss a beat. I had to go back to old text messages to jog my memory and piece it together with the story she told me while I was in the chair.

After a day or two of reflecting and journaling, I explained to her that I wasn't ready when I called her and told her I would let go of the Hair Therapy salon. I'm sorry that she was a victim of my thought process and all the different ideas I had. Maybe we could work together; maybe we could do this; maybe we could do that. I needed to call her once I was certain and sure that I was done.

I told her something I discovered, which is how I wrote about her in an old text. My texts wrote about her as a king and me as queen. I believe my frame of thought was that she was the OG—the leader—and I was following in her footsteps. I looked up to and respected her. Although I messed the transition up initially, I was grateful that she was in this space and the community over ten years later. This was not my destiny. I was merely holding this space and keeping it warm for her to do all she had done. We both were misty-eyed. She gave me a hug, and it was a beautiful moment.

I didn't know that I rubbed her the wrong way and couldn't believe some of the stupid things I said back then while I was distressed. She asked me if I could, would I still come back. I told her I no longer had any interest in running a salon business but would always have an interest in purchasing a commercial space and smiled.

April is for Issa 2024

For Issa's birthday, I took him to see the progress of our house. They had broken ground, and there wasn't much to see, but he was still excited. I wore my "Make my ancestors proud one dream at a time" shirt, and I smiled the biggest smile with my new hair. When we were done, I took him to see Miss A at the former Hair Therapy location. She said he looked like me; he was my twin. He looked around and said it was nostalgic to be there; he hadn't been in the space in so long. I reflected on how far we've come and how much has changed since he was a little boy.

There was a time when I wanted the dream so badly that I left my momma's house but didn't get my own apartment because I couldn't afford the expenses of running the business and having a home. For at least a year, I lived at my shop with my son, and he remembers portions of that. I bathed him in the utility sink. When he got a scratch from falling off a bike, I bathed him in coconut milk for a week. Was I unknowingly not only healing his scars but cleansing his soul?

Next, we headed to Beat the Bomb. We hung out with friends and did a really fun activity. If you cannot beat the bomb by the end, you get splashed with paint. I had no idea what I was doing; we certainly did not beat the bomb and were splashed with paint.

When we came home, I lit a little candle in his room that smelled good. His room was nice and clean. To give him positive energy, I sang Happy Birthday to him. We were singing it all day, and when we were done singing, lights flickered several times, and he said, "Grandma." It was a perfect ending to a fun and local day.

On April 6, we kept the fun going. I decorated the living room as usual with Spider-Man again, but this time with a different movie and schematics (mainly white and black). The cupcakes were red, and the gifts were wrapped in shiny red paper. He received his Jordan Reimagines, which made him feel even more like Spider-Man. The retro ones that Miles has in the movie are incredibly challenging to find. He was still very surprised and happy.

We set out to go to an indoor water park. He had way too much fun; he was running, slipped, and hit his head. I couldn't do anything but hold on to my heart. We capped off the celebration with a Sunday brunch at a DC vegan restaurant. Issa sat at the head of the table, and we cheered with juice and hot chocolate. The day would not have been complete if he hadn't gone to Gravelly Point to watch the planes. We watched those planes until he was super tired and ready to go home.

I spent the rest of the month supporting Issa and track. Practice was every day, and he did not win a race the entire season. His goal was to keep beating his personal best and get better. I could see the look on his face when he realized there would be times in life when everyone around you was bigger than you, faster than you, and stronger than you. The first lesson we learned is don't give up. Iron sharpens iron. I have no doubt that at some point, I will be watching my kid conquer the obstacle of not being able to win a race at a meet. It will take conditioning, discipline, and time.

I received a call saying that we would receive some money because Issa's dad was incarcerated and had to pay his child support to get out. I did think it was sad that his life had to be in danger for him to pay for Issa. But it was interesting to see how life can take care of things, and you do not have to be vindictive for it to happen.

In May, I screamed for joy as my friend became a doctor. The week before, her little sister graduated from George Mason University with a Bachelor's in global affairs—evidence of the impact of big sisters as a role model. I remember when she started the journey, and now she was done. Issa drew a special card with the logo of her university on it, and she loved it. We did the customary flowers, but this was big, so we had to go big and got her a watch. Movado's reminds me of my dad. And time reminds me of my grandfather. He says it's the most expensive thing on earth and never to waste it.

I loved the way she used her time, which was always efficient and impactful. She walked across the stage, newly married with a child and doctorate in hand. That's how you do it. So much in life can change in one year, and she was an example of letting nothing stop you. Let this story be a testimony: you do not have to suffer. It does not have to be bad; you do not have to try harder. When it's for you, it is obvious, and the actions are made to bring the story together. While I know sometimes people have houses and children, and it's all a sham, that's not what we're talking about here. We are talking about genuine respect and love for each other. A solid foundation built on knowing what to do when you meet a gem and something that feels good.

Grad season continued, and my dad visited because my cousin was graduating from Howard University to become a dentist. It was the season to be proud. He came to hang out with me and Issa for a few days. We took that opportunity to go to the house and see the progress. The framework was up, and Issa's new slogan was "sticks to bricks," although there was not a brick in sight.

I celebrated ten years of Hair Therapy. Although we didn't have sales going through the roof the way that I had imagined, something that we did have was valuable: community and sharing our knowledge with each other. I held this celebration in a nail salon, where we had a complete takeover for four hours. We all got manicures and pedicures. Our VIP room had a karaoke machine, and it was a good time. I presented my new product, Hair Therapy nail oil, to promote and encourage customers to use it on their nails. I told myself, *Something's gonna pop if you don't stop*," and I just kept coming up with ways to reinvent and rework what we already have.

It was time for the last concert with Issa's favorite chorus teacher. The family came out to support Issa in his first solo from *Hamilton*. He also received an award for being the first sixth grader to become a Seminole Singer. She told me, "Do not yell," and the first thing I did when she said his name was yell. I didn't know he was receiving an award. The kids were crying in the finale during the concert, and I was crying in the audience. I didn't know who would be their next leader, but it would be tough to fill her shoes. Issa presented her with flowers.

In an unforeseen turn of events, my son's math teacher didn't return to school. He was gone for two weeks, and I didn't suspect he was gone until Issa received a low score on a unit test. I inquired, and the school said they're not required to tell us they don't have a teacher for fourteen days. I thought this was absurd. I complained to the district about it. This still didn't solve the issue of Issa not having a teacher. I relied on my friend, Dr. Rufaro, who recently graduated, to regularly meet with me on Zoom to catch Issa up to speed. Dr. Rufaro helped Issa with his final math presentation. The requirement was to select a place to travel in the world, and the mathematical part involved breaking down the trip's expenses using charts and tables. We tried to get Issa to select something simple like Kings Dominion; instead, he chose Tokyo, where he could go drifting.

With my friend's support and a few sleepless nights, Issa raised his F in the fourth quarter. I named this series of study sessions Fourth Quarter on the Hair Therapy University page. I shared this link with the school, but I don't believe leadership shared it with the children because no one else logged on. I was able to help Issa's best friend because he lived down the street. It was a shame that so many kids were left behind.

It was the home stretch to summer break this year, and we missed no school days gallivanting around the world. We were dedicated to the mission. We were involved. I could not believe I turned into that track mom who took orange slices, chips, and water. I was out on the field. I'm the furthest thing from athletic. I am just an Issa enthusiast. Wherever he was, I wanted to be a stone's throw away. I made myself useful when one kid fell hard, and no one rushed to his aid. I disinfected his cut and wrapped it in gauze. I'm not sure how I did it. My knees were weak the entire time. I texted my nurse friend as though I was doing triple heart surgery.

That weekend, we let off some stress by going to the biggest bounce house. Apparently, it wasn't enough because I was still finding pieces of broken locs from Issa. I wrote to Rita about my concerns, and she sent articles she thought would help. Eventually, Issa attended hypnotherapy with her, and that solved the problem.

The Walkthrough

June 10. It was time for my construction walkthrough. It was sentimental; owners get to write something on the walls or floor before the walls go up. Issa wrote "Issa's room forever" on the floor. I wrote, "Candy did it; the family was here. Auntie Roxy, Uncle D, Issa, and me :) 2024." I wore my Hair Therapy shirt. I had teal and black hair and wore my teal glasses, smiling from ear to ear. It was hitting me that it was really going to happen.

Although, on the back end, they gave me hell about my salary. They miscalculated it, and I was kicked out of the first-time homeowner buyer program for making too much. I fussed and fought for my rights. Then I was told to adjust my salary to something lower than the inflated number, but it was still not accurate. That was annoying. Finally, the very last week before closing, what did they ask me? Adjust it to my actual fucking salary. I couldn't tell if this happened due to incompetence or one of those experiences that only happens when you're Black.

After our visit, Issa drew a portrait of himself from a selfie he took in his room. All I could do was stop and stare. The portrait looked just like him. His drawing skills were evolving. He said, "Mom, I did not know I could do this."

I encouraged him to practice more because if that's what he could do without knowing he could, imagine what would happen if he practiced. He also sketched the house. It made me smile. I love how he records things through drawings. The last thing I drew was Mickey Mouse in the ninth grade. I'm more into making floor plans. However, his dad is an extremely good artist, and his paternal grandfather was also. I think Issa's destined to be good at sketching forever.

We went to New York for our annual birthday and Father's Day combo in June. I celebrated my cousin's birthday painting in Harlem, and we also went to dinner, where they set her chicken on fire, which was really cool. We took Dad to a seafood place; he really enjoyed the seafood and lobster but ironically said the rice was better than everything. I don't know how to feel about rice being better than lobster, but as long as he smiled, that's all that mattered to me.

This month, a huge change took place in my life because my sister came from California to have much-needed surgery. This changed the house dynamics, and my peace became a stressful endeavor. Issa was excited to have a third person. He loved to scream *Hi auntie, Bye auntie, Hi auntie* every single time he saw her.

July was here; finally time to go on that trip SWG kept toying with. I had already gone with Issa, and now it was time for adult fun. I went with my aunty and coworker. We had a blast and chose to explore the North End of the beach. I hadn't been there before. The newer hotels are on that end. When I went with Issa, we stayed in a budget oceanfront suite, and it was perfect for that one-day getaway.

Since the ladies and I needed some R&R, I felt we needed a little luxury too. It was a tiny bit risky splurging before closing, but I had planned for it. My hair was in a yellow and black braided bob. I whipped out one of the sexiest dresses. It fit my body really well. There were a lot of comments when I posted it, and I put it with the Gwen Stefani song, "Luxurious." I was smiling and glowing because I knew I was on the cusp—I was almost there. Only a few people knew about the house. In the beginning, I was excited and slipped up, but I was sure to give no updates about it toward the end.

August 6 was my final walkthrough, and I saw the house complete for the first time. Issa was still chanting, "Sticks to bricks, sticks to bricks," and in three days. I would receive my keys.

On August 8, it was dark and raining. I lay in bed and my ears were ringing. I could not sleep. My son said, "Mom, there's a tornado watch." I said, "Of course there; is we are doing something big tomorrow. Whenever there's a big force of good, there's always something against it. Don't worry about it. Let's go to sleep to make sure we wake up on time."

On my way to signing on August 9, I really wanted to speak to my dad. I called to ask him how he was doing. He said he was fine. I told him that I had my Dubai pen and I couldn't wait to sign my documents with the pen he had given me since he wasn't there. When I arrived, My real estate agent friend was there to greet me with smiles. She opened the door, and we stood in the kitchen. I pulled out my pen. When I was told I couldn't use the pen because of its color, I was very upset, almost in tears. I called my dad and complained about it. I propped up my phone, and he watched me sign my photos with the pen they forced me to use.

When I was done, my sister took pictures, and my friend gave me flowers. It was nice. I was still working remotely, and after everyone left, I returned to work on the computer. My dad told me to call him when I was home at my mom's house.

Around 7 p.m., he asked, "Are you home yet?" I said, "No, what's going on?" He said, "It's Grandma; she died last night."

I asked my dad why he kept it from me, and he said he didn't want to ruin my big day. When my ears were ringing and I couldn't sleep, I knew something was wrong. I just couldn't figure out what. When I looked at ringing ears spiritually, it said it meant that an ancestor was trying to reach you. I couldn't understand why anyone was trying to reach me, and now I knew that my grandma was leaving.

I start rambling. "Dad. I'm sorry. Oh my gosh, what are we going to do? Does she have insurance; what are we going to do?" I was woeful. I told him I would tell Issa and call him back.

I called Issa downstairs, and he said in his little voice, "Yes, Mommy?" I couldn't look him in the face for one minute and not tell him what happened. "Baby, Great Grandma Marian is gone." He cried and he cried. I held him, and we cried together. The echoes of our cries bounced off of the walls of the empty house. He said, "Now I have no grandmas, no grandmas at all. By the time I grow up, no one will be here, and I will be all alone, Mom." I said, "We have a big family, that's not true, but Great Grandma outlived everyone. She was ninety-one, and it was her time; she was in pain."

Two hours later, he was playing his game. I looked at his resilience. He wasn't altogether better, but he also wasn't laid out on the floor. I thought that was admirable and interesting. I asked him if he wanted to leave. He said Grandma would want us to clean our new house, so that was what we did.

As the days went on, Dad and I talked about funeral arrangements. Things were moving really fast. I told him I would support whatever he chose to do. Upon reflection, since I had August 24 reserved for celebrating my birthday, I sent him a picture of my calendar. He called me right back and told me that the funeral was scheduled for August 24. My jaw dropped. I said, "Dad, is there a way we can change it? Is there no other day?" He told me when there's a death in the family, we have to make sacrifices. I felt my tears filling up, and I didn't know what to say. I said, "OK, Dad."

I called Rita and told her I didn't know why I felt so strongly about this, but I absolutely could not abandon this celebration. I'd been planning for a year; there had to be a way to honor my grandma without ignoring myself. She said, "You will have to apologize to your dad because you went straight into problem-solving and analysis and with not enough empathy for the pain he must feel. We will do your reading later and call upon your grandma to soften his heart, but it's very important that you apologize. Do it quickly before it is too late."

In my reading, Rita said that my dad's only thought was *My mom left me.* My grandma did not want me to cancel celebrations because she loved parties, and she planned to come. This is true. My grandma did it big on her birthday and went to Africa for one of her birthdays. Her seventy-fifth birthday was so big, everybody from the church came, and I remembered it for years.

I drove my car to Richmond, about an hour away from my house, to get a vegan Philly cheese steak for my nerves. I was so afraid to call my dad back. I called my dad back.

"Dad, I am so sorry for your loss and the pain you're experiencing right now. I didn't mean to be selfish or insensitive. It would mean so much to me if we could find another date; will you please consider it?"

He explained that my cousins were helping, and it also concerned their schedules and availability. We called them on three-way. My cousin asked if Saturday, August 24 was out of the question, and I confirmed. Then she proposed August 25. My goodness, it was the day after! Grateful that the date was moved, I said OK.

I proceeded to plan for the funeral and my birthday. I ordered things, cleaned, prepared, and organized. This was not just my birthday but a celebration of womanhood. With it in mind that my grandma's spirit would be present, I took one of her nightgowns and hung it in my closet. It was green and white. This way, her spirit would know she's in the right place.

SWG reached out and inquired about my birthday. Against my reservations, I agreed to let him take me out for my birthday. We went out on August 23. My dress was snakeskin, and my nails were lavish. He planned an eventful evening. We started with dinner. I promised myself to listen more than I spoke. The lobby had Black art and a nice atmosphere. I had the cauliflower steak, the lights were dim, and the place was sexy. Why was I sitting across the table from him after all of the work I had done? What the heck is wrong with me?

I asked him, "Why are we here?"

He said he just wanted to do something nice for me and had been thinking about me. I asked what exactly he was thinking about. He said he wondered what I was doing and how I was doing. I took the response at face value. When he asked me why I came, I told him that after all that had happened, I knew I could get good treatment from anywhere else, but the smaller person in me wanted him to do it. He said that was very honest.

We played mini-golf at a posh grown-up spot. Then we had a nightcap at one of my favorite vegan restaurants. At this spot, we were a bit close. He put his hand on my back, then attempted to put my hand on his.

I said, "No, you are showering me, and that is fine." Nothing in me wanted to put my hands on him because I understood now that my hands were healing. I felt strong enough that his touch wouldn't break me down. We shared dessert; it was so sweet.

The server said we were cute. We got compliments from people at the restaurant about how nice we looked together. I thought *We look like something because our fashion complements each other; it gives the perfect couple look.* People always asked how long we'd been dating and said stuff like, "Yes king, yes queen" when we walked. They don't know this man, and I was currently indifferent. Makes you wonder how many other nice-looking couples out there are the opposite of what they appear. Coordinating Air Maxes, matching Jordans, or matching pea coats cannot save you from being incompatible. We looked at her and simply said, "Thank you."

He wanted to know if I wanted to watch one of my favorite movies as a real nightcap. I told him you know neither of us would make it through a movie, and I needed to go home after. That was a defining moment I was proud of. I would have been right back where I started if I had gone back to his place. We sang out loud to R&B songs on the ride home, a fun first. I hugged him when he walked me to the door. We had a really good night, and I think that was the best last date ever. Under different circumstances, yeah.

Too much transpired for me to go back and feel that I would ever be safe. The fabulous evening was an ending I could live with. Did I miss kisses and sleeping in the same bed? Yes. Did I miss feeling like I was in competition with his ex and commitment was an issue? No. If ever there had been a time to lay it on thick with words to match the actions, that night would have been it. I did not hear him say, I can't sleep without you, and I'm ready for us for real. There was no ring in my pie. No declaration that the ex was out of the picture. I didn't hear the words, and I wasn't going to ignore that this time.

He also did not open my door at the beginning of the night. I didn't move until he did, but that's not the point. My dad has been opening the door for me since I was born. SWG had to be reminded to do that, and it wouldn't break his neck to do so. Some may say that is nitpicking. I think it is telling. I resumed being quiet after the date. I didn't want to use the outing as a segue for speaking all the time again. My birthday celebration was the next day, and as soon as he pulled off, I was in the kitchen cooking with my family. They teased me about my freak-um dress and asked how the date went.

My house reveal was a surprise to the attendees. I did not tell them the location was my home, and they slowly caught on one by one. I gave out the agenda in advance so everyone knew what to wear and the flow of the celebration. The color was green, the easiest color on the eyes. Color of inner peace and spiritual awakening, radiating tranquility. I made a welcoming continental breakfast spread. We had a coloring table for stress and conversation.

We opened the day with the sound bath from One with Ebony, and everyone present was free to participate. I saw many colors but mainly red and yellow. I had a masseuse in rooms one and two; bedroom three was a dedicated changing room. I shopped for weeks for mats, lotions, and orchids. Things that would be welcoming and unique to each bathroom in the house. Once the massages concluded, we hosted brunch for twenty-two people. My aunts, cousins, and I prepared the food ourselves. It was everything I thought it would be and more.

When it was time to sing Happy Birthday, I had an idea. Although I broke my back getting the perfect peridot green cupcakes from a very good vegan bakery, I wanted to use something else—the self-care candle that Dahlia brought me as a gift and presented during my first healing session at my mom's house. I had been waiting to use this candle. It had crystals, and I knew this was the perfect occasion. It was already on the table as a centerpiece. I was ready to stop coveting it and light it.

I gave my speech. I let everyone know they were important and valuable to my life, which is why I asked them to be there to share in this moment.

"Thank you for all the support you've given me over the years. Thank you for your dedication to healing individually, and I can't wait to see the power of what we can do collectively. Today is about peace. There is strength in numbers. We have been cleansing and purifying our home. That is why specialists are here to help us relax from the burdens of womanhood and motherhood. I see you and thank you for seeing me. Each wick on my candle represents me and my siblings. We are three without my mom. Thank you so much from the bottom of my heart for participating and being here with me today; moments like this cannot be duplicated."

I blew out my candles, they clapped, and I hugged everybody and felt a little teary. We broke all that sentimental mush with a mash-up of some birthday songs, starting with "Gracie's Corner" version.

I thought, *Grandma, you were so healthy and smart; thank you for showing me the way.* I was opening new doors in a peaceful and serene location with promising developments for the future. In that moment, I did not feel burdened. I felt chosen and grateful. *You knew that I finally figured out what I needed to do to take care of the family. You stayed here until you knew with confidence that this day would happen.* Not only will I maintain my house, but I vowed to maintain her legacy.

August 25. My sister, Issa, and I drove to New York for Grandma's funeral. Dad chose her emerald green dress as her final resting dress. I had green hair, and Issa had a green tie; we matched with Grandma one last time. Issa played his guitar acapella in front of Grandma's white casket, and he was one of the only people to volunteer to say a few words.

"My grandma was always old, so I didn't get to spend a lot of time with her. I love her, and I will miss her."

He made everyone laugh and cry. He was so strong; he was so brave. I don't believe in kids seeing open caskets or dead bodies, and my dad broke all kinds of traditions by keeping the casket closed for Issa, and I greatly appreciate him for that.

My dad did a wonderful job of delivering the eulogy that we wrote together. I sang verse one of "Lift Every Voice and Sing" and read verses two and three of the poem by James Weldon Johnson.

The repass was more like an after-party; people danced, and it was a true celebration of life. There were lots of food and pastries. I drove home that night with the intent to have Issa at school in the morning. When I crossed the Maryland border, all the emotions came from the soles of my feet, rushed their way up, and poured out of my eyes. *She is gone, she is gone, she is gone.* I wept and banged on the steering wheel, eventually using the steering wheel to lean on and sob into. My sister took over, and she got us home.

The upstairs of Grandma's house was recently damaged by tenants who abused it, making my childhood room unrecognizable and dingy brown. I spent the next weeks dedicated to finding professionals to restore Grandma's house. I worked collaboratively with my dad for weeks to bring the house into the 2024 desirable look. I wrote all the plans down. I did restoration everywhere. I gave my mom's house a facelift. After twenty years, it went from baby blue and beige to nautical navy and white. She would have loved that. A portion of Grandma's house is restored. It can build revenue to help our families sustain and stay in New York, which is a challenging and volatile market.

Per tradition, on August 28, 2024, I went to dinner with my son. My big boy and his button-up had a playlist for me. There was no kid bop on it; he had some solid selections ("Swang," by Rae Sremmurd, "Loop Hole," by Tee Grizzley, "Whiskey, Whiskey" by Moneybagg Yo, "Sicko Mode" by Travis Scott).

He made a card for me with a picture of the two of us and printed Happy Birthday on top. He decorated my room with café lights and ceiling water projection lights. He had a customized graphic of a cupcake with a candle, and the front read Happy 41st Birthday on the screen. Three lanterns were on my bed, and music was playing. I will never stop being googly-eyed and amazed when he makes mommy-specific gifts; they make me feel so special. He is getting older and mirroring the things I do for him. Evidence that children learn by observation.

The Rose

In this self-care September, I reflected on how quickly a year of no intimacy flew by. Thanks to a few things. The first was my rose. The second was having a goal that pushed me to my limits. I purchased my rose in February 2023. All that hot and cold, now I have someone to snuggle with, now I don't, had me stressed out. I needed something reliable. It had been years since I used any type of sex toy. I ordered two toys. One rose and one vibrator. I quickly learned that I don't enjoy sticking it to myself; I prefer to be stimulated by external pleasure.

The first time I tried the rose, the sensation was too much. I didn't understand how women were surviving it. Once the battery wore down and it was weaker, I found that to be better. Once I got the hang of it, I was a fiend. I wanted to rose myself to sleep every night I was not on my cycle. It significantly reduced the urge to text or talk to anyone from my past. I started experimenting with control. Testing if I could make myself climax quickly or if I could have some endurance. I even went so far as practicing which type of orgasm I wanted to have. Today, I would have a fast one. Today, I would have a medium orgasm. Today, I'd make my butt cheeks tremble and scream because I can't hold in how good the release is. I failed multiple times, barely making one minute with this intuitive sex toy. I also learned it was harder for me to have a big orgasm the first time but almost guaranteed the second time.

Also, what I thought about played a major role in how good the orgasm was. Many times, I reflected on my best sexual experiences. These reflections became less effective over time, and I whipped out my imagination for some pretty mean sex fantasies. For example, having their partner or exes watch them eat me out at gunpoint. Or an ex situationship of mine having to watch my new man have sex with me and be forced to suck his cum out of my pussy once he came. By gunpoint, of course. My outrageous porn imagination would send me to jail in real life. The concepts my mind created were crazy and mentally exciting but telling. I was definitely working through some resentment.

I left my sex-by-gunpoint era and had a no-men era. All my thoughts while rosing were about women, scissoring, strap-on sex, etc. If I even thought about a man, I would lose excitement. The next era was thinking about things I wanted, manifesting. That was new because who orgasms about reaching goals? I guess it's the same wheelhouse of men thinking about baseball so they could last longer. I thought about being on beaches and being happy. Jumping in waterfalls, building a big house that I designed on paper years ago. These orgasms had less guilt in them.

When I wasn't rosing, I was working on a goal that really pushed me to my limits. Preparing for the house required my income to be solid. The company I was with did advance pay every hour you worked, and when you were off, you were not paid. That is not a traditional pay system, and banks don't like nontraditional things. To be safe, I worked and took no days off, only a few hours as needed. I had only taken twelve hours off for the year, and it was September. They said I needed to take it due to federal regulations; that wasn't something I thought a job would ever tell me. I assured them I would be out of the office after closing.

Hustling to make money for RAE without using my tax refund was a goal. It was admirable that I had been pulling it off, but I didn't want to take away from my family during the year of responsibility. Chasing ticket sales and donors kept me busy. This was the first year I covered the expenses without personal sacrifice.

Keeping up with therapy for me and my son was a personal goal. He attended four appointments a month for talk therapy, plus phycologist appointments. Issa had been in therapy since 2018. He didn't like his first therapist and refused to open up to her. He loved his second therapist because he was a guy and was personable. He saw him from September 21, 2021 to February 15, 2023. Once he left the practice, the person Issa was referred to said she did not do televisits for kids. She insisted that they were not effective, and I had to make a choice: find someone new, stop therapy, or go in person. I was upset that she was uprooting a routine that worked for us but agreed to start in-person therapy on March 23. Once I added choir practice and track pick-ups, my life was picking Issa up or taking him somewhere five days a week from 2023 to 2024.

After a total of eight years for myself, my last therapy session was October 19, 2024. I saw my first therapist from 2012 to 2015. Sessions were primarily about postpartum and motherhood.

I dealt with shock and abandonment from 2012 to 2015. I had years of societal shaming, depression, and extreme anxiety but was told this is the norm by peers. Well, it didn't feel normal to me. I was told by the internet to choose better. Thank you, internet. It was here I learned to quiet the noise. I worked pretty hard at Hair Therapy. I created a space where I could think and be creative. Unfortunately, breaking even and no dental coverage caused health and fiscal stability problems.

The 2Pac era was from 2019 to 2024. *All Eyez on Me.* Me against the world. And an enormous number of family disagreements. Unrequited love. Lost hope to reconcile with my mom due to her passing. The emergence of acceptance was around 2021. The beginning of taking things less personally. The beginning of knowing when to leave. In 2023, concrete do's and don'ts were created. Friends were lost, and relationships dissolved. I was spreading myself thin trying to complete a million things, but that's something I had to work on by myself.

Eight years. I am so proud of myself; I am so proud of my son. He has his own therapy journey and works really hard on himself as well. Healed people hear differently and see differently. It feels so good to take deep breaths instead of shallow ones. I've built a community and learned how to ask for help. Cheers to a new chapter (era).

Year	Science/Therapy	Spiritual
2025		
2024	**Graduated Therapy**	One with Ebony – Intro to Sound Bath
	Dr Crosby	-Hypnotherapy
	Talk Therapy	-spiritual baths
2023	-Dating	-readings
		-new journal
		Rita (Hoodoo)
		-Readings -Soul Retrieval
		-Womb Repair -Meditation
		Dahlia (Reiki)
2022	-Family Dynamics	
2021	-Raising a kid with ADHD	
	-Career Strategy	
2020	-Covid-19 Coping	
2019	-Friendship Evaluation	
	-Unrequited Love	
2018	-Grief / Family Dynamics	One with Ebony – Intro to Thai
2017		
2016		
2015	**Graduated Therapy**	One with Ebony – Intro to Yoga
	Dr Salazar	
	Talk Therapy	
2014	-Ruminating Thoughts	
	-Mood Stabilization	
2013	-Parenting Techniques	
	-Meditation	
2012	-Mental Excercizes	

THIS STORY IS TOO LONG. WHAT ARE THE LESSONS?

1. I am strong enough to wait for the love that deserves me.
2. I am stronger than my anxiety.
3. I am confident things will work out even if I am struggling right now.
4. Always go to your regular nail tech before a vacation; no sub-techs.
5. Just because you have been doing well for a while does not mean you can't fuck up. Do not be overconfident; it is indeed a time to be more protective of your progress.
6. Ignoring the flags, your gut, and established outcomes from prior mistakes will lead you back to square one.
7. Please rest and remember the fire never lasts forever,
8. Life changes start with an application; complete them
9. Proximity and consistency are enough for a child to interpret what they are seeing as relationships.
10. Evaluate the level of commitment within some of your connections/relationships, whether they match your efforts, and if you want them to continue.
11. Your best opportunity is to allow those who only desire to take from you to help themselves while you're going through your healing process and making progress forward.
12. Seek to understand how others think while balancing that with speaking your truth.
13. Decisions should be based on your long-term future rather than any short-term gains of comfort and avoidance.
14. As you grow and expand, others will want to attach to that energy, and it will be up to you to use your discernment whether you allow it.

15. Anything or anyone that leaves you feeling disempowered should be released or allowed to move on from you.
16. Love does not fit within "should" and fixed presuppositions.
17. Get the help; if that doesn't work, get more help.
18. It is *never* a good idea to jeopardize your healing. Anything or anyone that is for you will be there after your session. There can be no bending or negotiating with yourself about this.
19. Call people back, visit people you care about; they can pass away any time.
20. Procrastination kills dreams.
21. Sometimes people come back into your life because time has passed, not because they have changed.
22. Stay away from anyone who is hung up on their ex; you will have his body, and she will have his heart. That's a bad deal.
23. A man who does not send you music does not like you (opinion).
24. Do not ignore what you already know. If you do not know, stop as soon as you figure it out.
25. Research current events of places you plan to visit, not just statistics on crime.

CONCLUSION

The journey of celibacy has been a wild ride. Celibacy is not mandatory for all, but it was important for me to experience. The synergistic effect between sex/sexual abuse and my self-esteem altered sound decision-making at times. I started the journey while I was in a place of great sorrow and loss. Even then, it was clear to me that not taking time to heal could result in ending the legacy of my mother, for myself, and make life for my son harder than it needed to be.

After years of building and completing to-do lists, I saw enormous progress. It wasn't until I let my guard down with the wrong person that I realized my fortress can be penetrated when I am not careful and open the door. I am not immune to making bad choices just because I've been making good ones for a while, and the quickest route to demise is ignoring what I already know. In therapy, we explored the brain; however, for my full recovery and to unlock my strongest will, I needed to explore my soul.

I didn't trust the process and I still went through it because it was the grand design of my life to do so. I admit that going through the process willingly and intentionally is a much better experience than being catapulted by a lesson. The circle of life has three stages: birth, life, and death. Customarily, you can't choose when you are born and when you die. However, you can choose how you live. My quality of life has improved significantly since I have gone inside of myself for the answers that were always there. Mistakes are disappointing, but they do not define me. It is never too late to get back on track and never too late to improve.

Some destinations will require me to fly, and I can't soar if I am being held down by the traumas of my past. My fuel is the vision of the future, and I have gained a profound appreciation for the present, knowing that each positive moment I have will become a fond memory.

Celibacy is often associated with a sacred religious vow, while abstinence is associated with restraining from something. I chose to address my journey as celibacy because of what it evolved into. A trauma-filled, fear-based response evolved into alignment and spiritual evolution. Looking from a deeper lens, one could say that breaking the abstinence and finding the strength to start over is where the real breakthrough took place. Now, I am celibate. I am consciously in tune with all that I am. I am aligned. I understand.

Four years and four months is specific. What is the spiritual meaning of four? Simply put, four represents stability and balance. It is connected with nature by representing all elements—earth, fire, wind, and water—which signify a cyclical rhythm. Historically, architects employed stability in their designs, such as the pyramids. http://planetnumerology.com

When I thought my world was falling apart, it was being restructured. I have a solid foundation, and whatever I build on top of it will be able to stand the test of time.

4.4 Playlist

4.4 Movies and Shows

4.4 Books

Dear Reader*,

As an immersive creator, listening to music can take me back in time. Music provides the feeling and the tone. If you are an immersive reader, I created a playlist for you. When it comes to movies and shows, there is always something we haven't heard or seen, and the community is shocked to hear it. The same is true with books. Sometimes, titles become popular, and we still don't read them (in my case, listen). I have extracted and created these lists for you as a reference point. They are indexed by the month and year I mentioned them.

Love Always,

Candalada

*Dear Reader is an ode to Bridgerton

4.4 Playlist

"I Will Always Love You" Whitney Houston – Sept 2018
"Candy" Cameo – Feb 2018
"With Me," "Too Deep," "Do it Well" DVSN – May 2018
"Body Smile," "Nuh Time/Tek Time" – DSVN 2018
"Waterfalls" LVNDVN – July 2018
"I Want You" Luke James – July 2018
"On Chill" Wale – Aug 2018
 "All the Kisses" Tammy Rivera – Aug 2018
"Hello" Erykah Badu – Dec 2019
"The Light" The Album Leaf Into The Blue Again – July 2022
"Teen Spirit" Nirvana – Nov 2022
"Anti-Hero" Taylor Swift – Jan 2022
"Under the Influence" Chris Browne – Jan 2023
"Luxurious" Gwen Stefani – July 20224
"Swang" Rae Sremmurd – Aug 2024
"Loop Hole" Tee Grizzley – Aug 2024
"Whiskey, Whiskey" Moneybagg Yo – Aug 2024
"Sicko Mode" Travis Scott – Aug 2024

Hymns and Spiritual

"Greet Somebody in Jesus' Name" Sept 2023
"Kumbaya" Sept 2023
"Love Lifted Me" Sept 2023
"Let Your Living Water Flow" Sept 2023
"Lift Every Voice" Sept 2023
"Amazing Grace" Sept 2023
"Let the Flowers Bloom Again" Sept 2023

4.4 Movies and Shows

Wreck-It Ralph 2 – Nov 2018
Bumblebee – Dec 2018

My Online Valentine – Feb 2019
Toy Story 4 – Oct 2019
The Secret Life of Pets 2 – Oct 2019
The Lion King – Oct 2019
Spider-Man Far from Home – Oct 2019
Hell's Kitchen – Oct 2019
Dora and *the Lost City of Gold* – Oct 2019
Preparatory – Nov 2019
In Time – Dec 2019
The Walking Dead – Jan 2020
The Photograph – Feb 2020
The Last Dance (ESPN) – May 2020
For Life (ABC) – May 2020
Little Fires Everywhere (Hulu) – May 2020
Ozark (Netflix) – May 2020
Becoming (Netflix) – May 2020
The Chi – Aug 2020
P-Valley –Aug 2020
Ramy – Dec 2020
Jingle Jangle – Dec 2020
Soul and Ma Rainey's Black Bottom – Dec 2020
Avengers: Endgame – Jan 2021
The Hunger Games – Jan 2021
Bridgerton – Feb 2021
Judas and the Black Messiah March – 2021
The United States vs. Billie Holiday March – 2021
The White Lotus – Sep 2021
The Sweet Life – Sep 2021
Mare of Eastown – Sep 2021
50 First Dates – Jan 2022
Coming to America – March 2022
Spike Lee's Do the Right Thing – March 2022
Malcolm X – March 2022

Woman King –Sep 2022
Harriet – March 2023
Transformers: Rise of the Beast – June 2023
Spider-Man Across the Spider-Verse – June 2023

4.4 Books and Poems

Becoming by Michelle Obama – Nov 2018
Black Rice by Judith Carey – June 2020
The Mis-Educated Negro by Carter G. Woodson – July 2020
The Souls of Black Folk by W.E. Dubois" – Oct 2020
Beautiful Reject by Candalada – Feb 2021
Breaking Night by Liz Murray – Oct 2021
Beautiful Reject Coloring Book by Candalada– Feb 2024
Lift Every Voice and Sing by James Weldon Johnson – Aug 2024

ACKNOWLEDGMENTS

To my mother, Shelly B., you are missed. I was so perplexed about our relationship as a teen. As I become more seasoned in my motherhood journey, I understand you more each day. I understand why you got straight to the point when you spoke. I see why you enjoyed staying in rather than going out. Being a mom is demanding. I am grateful for all that you have done for me. Thank you for creating me. I love you.

To my dad, Dale H., thank you for always telling me I can do anything. No one understands me more than you. How do you do that? It's magical. I have enjoyed traveling with you these past few years, and I will cherish those moments forever.

To my inner child, may you always feel protected and loved.

To my siblings, I encourage you to go deep within. Every experience you have shapes who you are.

To my family, I am eternally grateful for my Aunt Roxanne who, every time I told a story, would say, "Girl, you should write a book; when you describe things, I can see them so clearly." I admire your confidence, and I value your support through the years.

To my heartbeat, my son. Your birth was pivotal; everything in me has changed since your creation. If my only purpose in life was to create you, I am fulfilled. Your existence placed me on a quest to reflect on all I have done and figure out how to be the best version of myself. As you grow up, I will ensure you have a mom who is mindful and supportive rather than bitter, broken, and wounded. You are my *why*.

To my mentor, Dr. Davis, I've watched you contribute to several books and publish educational books. You provided an example of how to use education as a tool to solve simple and complex issues. While this book is not of the same nature and genre as your work, the foundation and examples you laid before me were impactful and inspiring. Thank you for encouraging my business and creative endeavors without placing a higher value on one side over another.

To Dr. Salazar, your decorum is unmatched. You were my introduction to therapy, and I was so blessed to have you as my first experience. You saved me from myself. Your cognitive exercises helped me overcome intrusive thoughts. You are a gem to the world.

To Dr. Crosby, thank you for showing me that even with a "big, beautiful mind," it is always OK to simplify and be effective. Thank you for being a listener and teacher. I enjoy your combined usage of self-experience, scientific modules, and real-world solutions (enrollment in helpful programs). Knowing you has improved my mental health and quality of life.

To my Hair Therapy family. Thank you for allowing me to grow personally and professionally. Thank you for trusting me; the shop is the home of all relationship tea. We have shared some of life's biggest milestones, graduations, prom, over-the-hill parties, marriages, and new home purchases. You are my extended family. Special thanks to Mrs. Matthews and Dr. Groff for believing in and investing in me.

To my photographer, Kevin Marable. You are light. You are patient and inciteful. I admire your relentless drive and your passion for creating.

To One With Ebony, thank you for your patience and kindness over the years. I have seen you blossom from drop-in classes to international retreats. You are walking in your purpose, positively impacting those around you and the center of your tribe.

To Dahlia, you magical, powerful being. You are a wonder and a real OG. Thank you for breaking the thick layers of chaos and opening the portal of communication between myself and me, thus making it easier for others to work with me and go further than I have ever been before. Thank you for identifying my gifts and allowing me the time and the space to figure out who and what I am. Thank you for your organization and presenting things in written form to be discovered later.

To A. Ryze, thank you for adorning my body with your art for two very important occasions in my life: the memorial of my mother and the release of *Beautiful Reject: The Coloring Book Cognitive Distortions.* Thank you for sharing your sweetest tone to speak to your kids and my soul. Thank you for referring me to Rita. She has been a major part of my awakening and progress.

To Rita, thank you for sharing your gifts and pouring your love onto not only me but my son, Prince Issa. Thank you for exploring our minds and our souls and placing protection over our lives. Thank you for being love itself.

Thank you for using your energy to help repair and restore the Hopkinson and Browne legacies.

To my ex-situationships, you were a catalyst, and for that, I say thank you.

Finally, to my editor, Wendy Hall. I value your knowledge and skills. I am blessed to have connected with you. Your knowledge and professionalism have been the key to refining my creative and wildly unstructured writing. I love your feedback. You make me better.

Thank you.

ABOUT THE AUTHOR

Candalada is the founder of Hair Therapy, a beauty consulting company. She is a former instructor of Business Communication at Shenandoah University's School of Business and has more than ten years of digital media experience. She obtained her Bachelor's in Mass Communication, with a concentration in Media Studies and a minor in Business Administration at Shenandoah University. She attended Trinity Washington University for a Master's in Mass Communications with a concentration in Political Rhetoric.

Former President Barack Obama presented the President's Volunteer Service Award to Candalada for her special service commitment to economic opportunity. She was raised in Brooklyn, New York, and born to parents from Guyana, South America. Candalada lives in Northern Virginia with her son.

BIBLIOGRAPHY

https://thejoywithin.org/empowerment-exercises/

automatic-writing

https://www.intuitivejournal.com/what-is-clairsentience/

https://spiritualityessence.com/spiritual-meanings-of-alchemists/

https://www.britannica.com/dictionary/clairvoyance

https://www.poetryfoundation.org/poems/46549/lift-every-voice-and-sing

Beautiful Reject 7 Years of Delusional Dating by Candalada pg. 13

https://www.whatspiritual.com/spiritual-meanings-of-color-green/

https://jamaica-gleaner.com/article/news/20181202/religion-culture-hoodoo-life-saving-magic-southern-slaves

https://www.nps.gov/articles/000/hoodoo-in-st-louis-an-african-american-religious-tradition.htm

NOTES

Made in the USA
Columbia, SC
07 March 2025